# CRITICAL THINKING AND CLINICAL REASONING IN THE HEALTH SCIENCES:
## AN INTERNATIONAL MULTIDISCIPLINARY TEACHING ANTHOLOGY

NOREEN C. FACIONE, PH.D.    PETER A. FACIONE, PH.D.

© 2008 NOREEN C. FACIONE & PETER A. FACIONE
ALL RIGHTS RESERVED.
PUBLISHED BY THE CALIFORNIA ACADEMIC PRESS LLC, MILLBRAE, CA
WWW.INSIGHTASSESSMENT.COM

ISBN: 1-891557-60-2
ISBN-13: 978-1-891557-60-6

© 2008 Noreen C. Facione and Peter A. Facione

All rights reserved. No part of this book may be reproduced in any form by Photostat, microfilm, PDF, email, internet, retrieval system or any other means, without the written permission of the authors.

The editors may be contacted through the publisher, The California Academic Press LLC.

>    The California Academic Press
>    217 La Cruz Avenue
>    Millbrae, CA. 94030
>    United States of America

>    Front and Back Cover designs and cover art
>    2008 © Measured Reasons LLC, Hermosa Beach CA

>    ISBN: 1-891557-60-2
>    ISBN-13: 978-1-891557-60-6

Printed in the United States of America

>    10 9 8 7 6 5 4 3 2

# Contents

| | |
|---|---|
| Preface | vi |
| List of Authors | vii |
| "Critical Thinking and Clinical Judgment,"<br>    Noreen C. Facione & Peter A. Facione | 1 |
| "Interpreting Benevolence and Righteousness in<br>    Contemporary Health Care,"<br>    Agnes Tiwari & K. H. Yuen | 15 |
| "Nurturing Students' Meta-Cognition and Self<br>    Reflection Through On-line Journaling,"<br>    Carol Giancarlo-Gittens | 25 |
| "Developing On-Line Cases for Teaching Critical<br>    Thinking and Clinical Reasoning Skills,"<br>    Sara Kim, *et. al.* | 45 |
| "An Analytical and Evaluative Approach to<br>    Community-Based Cancer Screening and<br>    Prevention projects," Noreen C. Facione | 55 |
| "Advocating through the Media: Cultivating CT<br>    Dispositions in a Distance Learning Course,"<br>    Mary M. Hoke & Leslie K. Robbins | 67 |
| "Unfolding Case Studies: Dynamic Mental Models in a<br>    Public Health Context," Jo Azzarello | 75 |
| "Roleplay Strategies for Critical Thinking in<br>    Psychiatric Mental Health," Tim Blake | 85 |
| "Keeping a Journal of Reflections on Learning,"<br>    Anna Chur-Hansen | 93 |
| "Teachable Moments in Clinical Practice: Promoting<br>    Clinical Judgment Skills," Margot Thomas | 101 |
| "The Clinical Sieve: a Visual Implement to Share the<br>    Diagnostic Thinking," Carlos A. Cuello-García | 109 |
| "Using Short Cases to Teach Thinking,"<br>    Marilyn H. Oermann | 123 |
| "A Case Study Tutorial with a Guided Reasoning<br>    Method to Develop Self Evaluation of Critical<br>    Thinking and Clinical Reasoning Skills,"<br>    Wolter Paans, *et. al.* | 131 |

| | |
|---|---|
| "Promoting Cognitive and Metacognitive Thinking Skills by Reflecting with Self-Regulated Learning Prompts," Ruth Anne Kuiper | 145 |
| "Prioritizing Nursing Assessments and Care," Susan Sandstrom | 155 |
| "Teaching Critical Thinking in Medicine: A Journey Back to the Future," Milos Jenicek | 163 |
| "Reflection on Practice: A Workshop Exercise," Kathleen Chirema | 179 |
| "Evaluating a Nutritional Supplement with SOAP Notes to Develop CT Skills," Greg A. Brown | 189 |
| "From 'What' to 'Why' – Reflective Storytelling as Context for Critical Thinking," Susan Forneris and Sue Ellen Campbell | 203 |
| "The Poster: A Critical Thinking and Creative Strategy in a Research Course ," Joanne Profetto-McGrath | 213 |
| "Problem-Based Learning in a Competency-Based Medical Assistants Curriculum," Rodney L. Tomczak | 221 |
| "Using Theoretical Foundations for a Community Health Nursing or Population Health Course," Caroline R. Ellermann | 231 |
| "Preparing Overseas Nurses to Work in Australia," Lee Huang Chiu & Meng Lim | 241 |
| "Thinking Critically About the Care of Patients with Neurological Disorders," Kyung Rim Shin | 249 |
| "Using the Creative Arts to Develop Critical Thinking Skills: Examining the Qualitative Method of Ethnography," Beth P. Velde | 257 |
| "Working with Patients Who Self-Harm," Margaret McAllister | 267 |
| "Training the Discovery of Evidence of Critical Thinking," Peter A. Facione | 279 |

# Preface

When objective measures reveal weaknesses in reasoning skills and habits of mind, what can we do to strengthen those skills and to foster more positive dispositions? This question, phrased in different ways perhaps by supervisors, educators, and other concerned professionals, has become a frequent refrain over the past fifteen years. It is a good question – an honest and concerned response to the variances in health science practitioners' and students' critical thinking skills and dispositions manifested in both reasoning test scores and in practice behaviors.

We are learning more about how humans actually try to understand problems and how they actually make judgments. Perhaps more importantly, we are learning more about how they make bad judgments, often without realizing it. In Chapter 1 we provide a survey of some of the new conceptualizations about the human judgment process, and position this collection of best practices as addressing the more reflective and deliberate thinking processes involved in clinical judgment. This component of the human reasoning process, the effort to make a purposeful and reflective judgment, has been referred to as critical thinking.

We have long advocated active learning techniques. The skillful use of problem-based learning, case studies, think-aloud, reflective logs, role-play, team problem-solving, and similar educational approaches have been demonstrated to be more successful in engaging students in the exercise of their skills in interpretation, analysis, inference, evaluation, explanation, and meta-cognition. The research on teaching methods in the health sciences and beyond shows too that active learning pedagogies foster and sustain positive habits of mind such as truth-seeking, inquisitiveness, open-mindedness, maturity of judgment, and confidence in reasoning. The positive effects of these approaches have registered as significant improvements in students' reasoning test scores and have been documented in the health sciences educational research literature in growing numbers of publications over the past decade or more.

Happily, conversations mired in the false dichotomy of "content vs. process," smothered by a defensiveness blaming the students or assailing the testing instruments, or clouded by a naiveté which rails against objective testing, are becoming more and more passé. The concern has become specific and practical: What can I do in my classes to improve my students' reasoning test scores and their clinical judgment processes?

This anthology offers some answers by way of successful examples of favorite lessons which work when teaching for both thinking and content. The authors in this anthology work in health sciences professional development and education. All of them have published their educational research. They are drawn from a broad spectrum of health sciences professions, professional levels, and academic ranks. From four different continents, they represent both pre-service and in-service programs. We sincerely thank these fine authors for working with us to be able to share what they have learned with you.

Noreen & Peter Facione<br>
Hermosa Beach, California, 2008

# Author List

Jo Azzarello, Ph.D., RN. College of Nursing, Oklahoma Health Sciences Center, Oklahoma City, Oklahoma, USA

Tim Blake, MS, RN. School of Nursing, Ohio University at Zanesville, Zanesville Ohio, USA

Doug Brock, Ph.D. School of Medicine, University of Washington, Seattle, Washington, USA

Greg A. Brown, Ph.D. Exercise Science, University of Nebraska, Lincoln Nebraska, USA

Sue Ellen Campbell, Ph.D., RN. Department of Nursing, College of St. Catherine, St. Paul, Minnesota, USA

Kathleen Chirema, Ed.D. School of Human and Health Sciences, University of Huddersfield, Queensgate, West Yorkshire, United Kingdom

Lee Huang Chiu, D.Ed. School of Nursing and Midwifery at Victoria University, Melbourne City, Victoria, Australia

Anna Chur-Hansen, Ph.D. Department of Psychiatry, Royal Adelaide Hospital, University of Adelaide, Adelaide SA, South Australia

Carlos A. Cuello-García, MD. School of Medicine, Instituto Tecnológico y de Estudios Superiores de Monterrey, Monterrey, Mexico

Caroline R. Ellermann, Ph.D., RN. School of Nursing, Northern Arizona University, Flagstaff, Arizona, USA

Noreen C. Facione, Ph.D., FAAN. Professor Emerita, School of Nursing, University of California San Francisco, California, USA

Peter A. Facione, Ph.D. Professor of Philosophy and Provost, Retired, Loyola University Chicago, Chicago Illinois, USA

Susan Gross Forneris, Ph.D., RN, CRRN. Department of Nursing, College of St. Catherine, St. Paul, Minnesota USA

Carol Giancarlo-Gittens, Ph.D. Director of Assessment, Faculty in Liberal Studies and Education, Santa Clara University, Santa Clara, California, USA

Tom Gallagher, MD. School of Medicine, University of Washington, Seattle, Washington, USA

Mary M. Hoke, Ph.D., RN. School of Nursing, New Mexico State University, Las Cruces, New Mexico, USA

Milos Jenicek, MD., Ph.D. Fellow of the Royal College of Physicians and Surgeons of Canada, Department of Clinical Epidemiology and Biostatistics, Michael de Grotte School of Medicine, McMaster University, Hamilton, Ontario, Canada

Sara Kim, Ph.D. School of Medicine & School of Dentistry, University of Washington, Seattle, Washington, USA

RuthAnne Kuiper, Ph.D., RN. School of Nursing, University of North Carolina, Wilmington, North Carolina, USA

Meng Lim, Ph.D., RN. School of Nursing and Midwifery at Victoria University, Melbourne City, Victoria Australia

Margaret McAllister, EdD. School of Health and Sport Sciences, University of the Sunshine Coast, Maroochydory DC, Queensland, Australia

Rose Nieweg, MScN, University Groningen and Kairos-Valeo Rotterdam in, The Netherlands

Peggy Odegard, Pharm.D., CDE, BCPS, School of Pharmacy, University of Washington, Seattle, Washington, USA

Marilyn H. Oermann, Ph.D., RN, FAAN, College of Nursing, Wayne State University, Detroit, Michigan, USA

Wolter Paans, MSc, RN. Hanze University Groningen and Kairos-Valeo Rotterdam in, The Netherlands

Joanne Profetto-McGrath, Ph.D., RN. Faculty of Nursing, University of Alberta, Edmonton, Alberta, Canada

Carolyn Prouty, DVM. School of Medicine, University of Washington, Seattle, Washington, USA

Leslie K. Robbins, DNS., RN. School of Nursing, New Mexico State University, Las Cruces, New Mexico, USA

Lynne Robins, Ph.D. School of Medicine, University of Washington, Seattle, Washington, USA

Susan A. Sandstrom, RN, MSN. School of Health Professions, College of Saint Mary, Omaha, Nebraska, USA

Sarah Shannon, Ph.D., RN. School of Nursing, University of Washington, Seattle, Washington, USA

Kyung Rim Shin, Ed.D., RN. FAAN, President of the Korean Nurses Association, Dean of the College of Health Sciences, and Vice President of Ewha Womans University, Seoul, South Korea

Margot Thomas, MScN, CNCCP, Pediatric Intensive Care, Children's Hospital of Eastern Ontario, Ontario, Ottawa, Canada

Agnes Tiwari, PhD, RN. Department of Nursing Studies, The University of Hong Kong, Hong Kong, China

Rodney L. Tomczak, DPM, Ed.D., American Institute of Alternative Medicine, Columbus, Ohio, USA

Frans van der Werf, MA, University Groningen and Kairos-Valeo Rotterdam in, The Netherlands

Beth P. Velde, Ph.D. Occupational Therapy, Assistant Dean College of Allied health Sciences, East Carolina University, Greenville, North Carolina, USA

Marleen Vermeulen, MScN, University Groningen and Kairos-Valeo Rotterdam in, The Netherlands

K. H. Yuen, PhD, Department of Nursing Studies, The University of Hong Kong, Hong Kong, China

# Critical Thinking and Clinical Judgment

## *Noreen C. Facione & Peter A. Facione*

Lives depend on competent clinical reasoning. Thus it is a moral imperative for health care providers to strive to monitor and improve their clinical reasoning and care related judgments. Knowing that this is the agreement owed to the public trust, agencies responsible for the accreditation of professional training programs and for the oversight of health care delivery have mandated the need to demonstrate competence in clinical reasoning in health care clinicians and students. This focus on competent reasoning and problem solving is not unique to health care. Sparked by a meeting of the United States Governors in the late 1980's, educational mandates to teach and assess thinking and problem-solving have become increasingly pervasive. In this effort, the health sciences and military science have led the way. Nearly all performance based credentialing programs and performance based funding initiatives require thinking and problem solving as one of the educational outcomes worthy of assessment (Ackerman, Rinchuse, & Rinchuse, 2006). This focus on assessing competence in reasoning and problem-solving is also becoming a standard in the workplace.

**The language of thinking**
Critical thinking and reflective problem-solving are two common terms for the cognitive processes involved in clinical reasoning. Excellence in professional judgment is the result of the sound use of critical thinking skills and the reliable and strong disposition to use those critical thinking skills. The alternative (acting without adequate analysis of the problem, repeating a previous care delivery behavior unreflectively, or continuing to carry out a care delivery behavior without evaluating its effect) is not a standard of practice any of us would uphold. The discussion below outlines what has been learned to date about how humans engage high risk problems and arrive at competent judgments about what to believe and what to do. It also explores the challenge we face as researchers and educators to facilitate improvements in clinical reasoning for ourselves, our students and our peers.

There are many prior accounts of the development of a consensus description of critical thinking, research carried out as a Delphi Study in the late 1980's (American Philosophical Association, 1990). and replicated by an independent study at Penn State University (Jones & Ratcliff, 1993). We recommend that those unfamiliar with this literature seek out any of these previous papers

(Facione & Facione, 1996a; 2006; Facione, Facione & Giancarlo, 2000). All of our work in instrument development and in the theoretical and practical study of human reasoning stems from this seminal study focused on the importance of everyday competence in reasoned judgment. Here we offer a brief overview integrating our research on defining and measuring evidence of everyday reasoning and judgment with the emerging consensus of research attempting to explain human reasoning processes. The result is informative for training critical thinking and clinical reasoning.

We begin with a definition of critical thinking derived from a consensus of disciplines, and used widely to ground teaching and assessment of critical thinking:

> "Critical thinking is the process of purposeful, self-regulatory judgment. This process gives reasoned consideration to evidence, contexts, conceptualizations, methods, and criteria." (American Philosophical Association Delphi Report, 1990).

In other words, critical thinking is a judgment process. Its goal is to decide what to believe and/or what to do in a given context, in relation to the available evidence, using appropriate conceptualizations and methods, and evaluated by the appropriate criteria. One way of describing how critical thinking relates to clinical judgment would be: *Critical thinking is the process we use to make a judgment about what to believe and what to do about the symptoms our patient is presenting for diagnosis and treatment.* This language is discipline free, because it refers to cognitive capabilities that can be generalized to all problem frames and all situational contexts. Here our interest is applying this terminology to the health sciences. To arrive at a judgment about what to believe and what to do, a clinician should consider the unique character of the symptoms (evidence) in view of the patient's current health and life circumstances (context), using the knowledge and skills acquired over the course of their health sciences training and practice (methods, conceptualizations), anticipate the likely effects of a chosen treatment action (consideration of evidence and criteria), and finally monitor the eventual consequences of delivered care (evidence and criteria).

**Adequate time to think**

Newell (1990) provided us with some concrete data on how long it actually takes to process a novel observation or a novel problem demanding of a response. When humans are queried on a novel issue or problem they require eleven to sixteen seconds to interpret the situation at hand and formulate even the most rudimentary reflective response. With forewarning they can summon relevant memories and content knowledge to inform their response, but otherwise processing time is required. Humans also frequently rely on heuristic maneuvers in an attempt to optimally address high stakes issues. Heuristic reasoning is believed to be most prevalent in time limited situations that do not admit of more reflective thinking, and in uncertain contexts when reflective thought fails to resolve ambiguities in the direction of a seemingly certain judgment (Gilovic, Griffin & Kahneman, 2002). More on this topic in the section below entitled 'Two systems of reasoning' but for now we return to the issue of 'time to think.'

Sixteen seconds is far longer than we are accustomed to waiting for a response after we pose an important question to a clinician, or even a student who is supposed to be prepared for the clinic. Both may feel the desire to respond thoughtfully and provide the optimal opinion, but far more often they first feel the pressure to respond quickly. So, what is forthcoming usually begins as only half-thought-out, with late breaking insights and necessary edits coming later as additional ideas are formulated. If the problem we pose is novel, and the clinician values accuracy and comprehensiveness as a component of the response, we may hear, "Now let me think about that for a moment." Hearing this response should engender confidence, but often instead it engenders doubt.
Learning to 'think aloud,' supplying evidence of the process of one's thinking and subsequent judgment (the assumptions made, the evidence base applied, the logical framing) offers a way for the listener to both evaluate the quality of the judgment and to learn to reason better themselves, This is demonstrated in discussions of think aloud exercises in some of the chapters to follow.

The accuracy of Newell's findings (the need for time to think) can be readily observed by asking anyone a novel question that requires reflective thought, and recording the time to a response. This is true regardless of expertise level, when the question or problem is truly novel. The physiological realities of human thinking make it important for educators to control the tempo of teaching and learning sessions if they are to effectively lead to improved clinical reasoning. Those who answer too quickly may have not thought well.

## Clinical reasoning and expertise

When clinical problems are familiar we can rely on externally developed protocols and internal 'mental scripts' to assist us in deciding what to believe and what to do about the problem. The externally developed protocols are elaborate and rise to the status of standards when the consequences of error are high and society is concerned with safety. There is still need for reflective thought when using protocols to assure that they are remain appropriate to the case and that expected results occur.

Internally developed 'mental scripts' are a function of expertise. The Dreyfus and Dreyfus model of expertise, which has been adapted by Benner for Nursing, (Benner 1994, 2004) is a phenomenological model that provides a description of the increasing sense of ease experienced over time by the clinician, moving from novice practice to more expert practice. Most models of expertise describe the novice who encounters a problem as attending indiscriminately to data in an attempt to recognize key relationships that will then allow the application of knowledge they believe to be relevant. The expert, in contrast, recognizes most problems by pattern, and resolves them without a significant awareness of reflective thinking. An expert does this through the retrieval of similar cases examples stored in episodic memory, a larger array of relevant knowledge stored in semantic memory, and the use of other heuristic thinking processes.

Benner's work describing the 'lived experience' of clinical reasoning notes the seeming inability to reflect on the thinking process that occurs in the expert clinician, describing it as 'intuiting.' In contrast, other cognitive science models of human reasoning explain this lack of conscious reflection as a function of several cognitive processes: heuristic reasoning (thinking maneuvers and shortcuts discussed below), automatic thought (the ability to accomplish an array of tasks without conscious attention), and the absence of perception of meta-cognition (listening to or thinking about your thinking). In the case of automatic thinking, familiarity with the tasks required frees cognitive resources to focused more specifically on only the unique aspects of the situation or perhaps even a different problem altogether. Recall the experience of driving home from work rehearsing approaches to resolving an interpersonal issue. Possibly you exit the car realizing that you really didn't 'see' the road and the other drivers for the majority of the thirty-minute drive. We even have language for this, 'running on autopilot.' But clearly some cognitive process, outside of your awareness, was monitoring your driving, making lane changes, braking, using turn signals, seeing the other cars. It is not known how often the autopilot function impacts clinical reasoning, nor what percentage of those impacts are negative.

Models of expertise help us to understand how different groups of clinicians are likely to approach clinical problems. A high level of expertise does not assure flawless reasoning in the clinician, any more than we can be sure frequent errors will be made by the novice. Novices are known to be slower to come to a judgment because they require more time for reflective thought and additional data searching. Novices err through problem misidentification and uncertainty about knowledge application. But experts also err due to problem misidentification, and they are more prone to being inattentive to those differences in the problem which make it the odd exception to the pattern and which render the modal responses inappropriate.

Understanding the cognitive effort entailed by the novice or expert state suggests several things about the training of clinical reasoning. Feelings of comfort when working on familiar problems in familiar contexts should not be confused with genuine clinical expertise. A person may be comfortable doing roughly the same thing over and over again, as demanding as that may be, but not have the expertise to be able to resolve new problems, to adapt old ways to new situations, or even to recognize limitations or shortcomings in the way he or she has always gone about doing those familiar things.

Expert clinicians are never beyond the need to actively monitor the soundness of their clinical reasoning. While we might allow ourselves to fold the laundry or cut the grass automatically, we can't allow this type of disconnect when the life or health of others is at stake. Hence, we need to continuously build the cognitive skills and habits of mind inherent in critical thinking as the preferred tools of the clinical judgment process, the conscious reflection about what to believe and what to do in the clinical context. Novice clinicians will have far more novel problems to address, but those who have stronger critical thinking skills will progress toward higher levels of competence and expertise.

**Two systems of reasoning**

Newer research in human reasoning finds evidence of the function of two interconnected 'systems' of reasoning. 'System 1' is conceptualized as reactive, instinctive, quick, and holistic. System 1 often relies on highly expeditious heuristic maneuvers which can yield useful response to perceived problems without recourse to reflection. By contrast, 'System 2' is described in the cognitive science literature as more deliberative, reflective, analytical, and procedural. System 2 is generally associated with reflective problem-solving and critical thinking. In its decision making processes System 2 also uses some heuristic maneuvers. We offer a fuller discussion in *Thinking and Reasoning in Human Decision Making: The Method of Argument and Heuristic Analysis*, (Facione & Facione, 2007) but will recap key elements here.

In humans these two systems never function completely independently. One is not naturally "better" than the other; in fact there are situations where each offers something of a corrective effect on the other. Because both systems rely on cognitive heuristics and because these maneuvers are known to have the potential to introduce error and biases into human reasoning, knowing something about heuristic reasoning is important to those who are attempting to train or to measure clinical reasoning. There is a growing literature on this research but reading several of the foundational books and papers will provide the needed insight into how we believe humans actually think and make clinical judgments (Gilovic, Griffin & Kahneman, 2002; Kahneman, Slovic & Tversky, 1982; Montgomery 1998). Here we provide only the briefest overview.

Some hypothesize that lacking claws, fangs, skeletal armor, protective fur, poisonous secretions, natural camouflage, strength, or speed, the human species survived, because of some other evolutionary advantage. One factor was the fast, efficient, and effective problem-solving made possible by heuristic reasoning. When used well, heuristic thinking helps us survive, but misuse of this type of reasoning, when not overridden by reflective thought (System 2), leads to predictable error. For example, consider the influence on behavior of the affect heuristic. This heuristic might function well pre-consciously like this: "unprotected needle –> BAD! (stop)" Twenty years after the AIDS epidemic, no reflective argument should be needed for a trained clinician to recognize the immediate danger presented by an unshielded needle. A misuse of this heuristic might be "comfort food –> GOOD," depending on how much one is trying to lose weight. Favoring choices that avoid loss, recognizing similarities, guessing about future events by playing a movie in your head of what will happen, and assuming one is able to control all threats, are examples of heuristic maneuvers that are typically below the level of conscious thought. This system 1 thought has a powerful effect on behavior as documented in these references here and others the end of this chapter. (Montgomery, 1998; Tversky & Kahneman, 1973; Kahneman, Slovic & Tversky, 1982; Weinstein, 1982).

Perhaps the current preoccupation with heuristic reasoning results from being relatively unaware of it in the past. While cognitive and social psychology has been working to impact the understanding of human reasoning, many have been holding to early descriptions by Plato and Aristotle of humans as always striving to be deliberative, reflective, and logical. Not true. Even when we are making high stakes clinical judgments, this is not true. The current conceptualization of two interacting and complementary systems better explains the evolutionary success of our species. A new method of argument analysis has emerged that includes an examination of the entire decision-making process, both System 1 and System 2 and the influences of cognitive heuristics along with argument making on decision outcomes (Facione & Facione, 2007). It's likely that this method of decision analysis will bring new insights about how some common clinical errors occur. The important thing to realize is that although you may not as yet have heard much about this in the past, this is how we think. Effectively

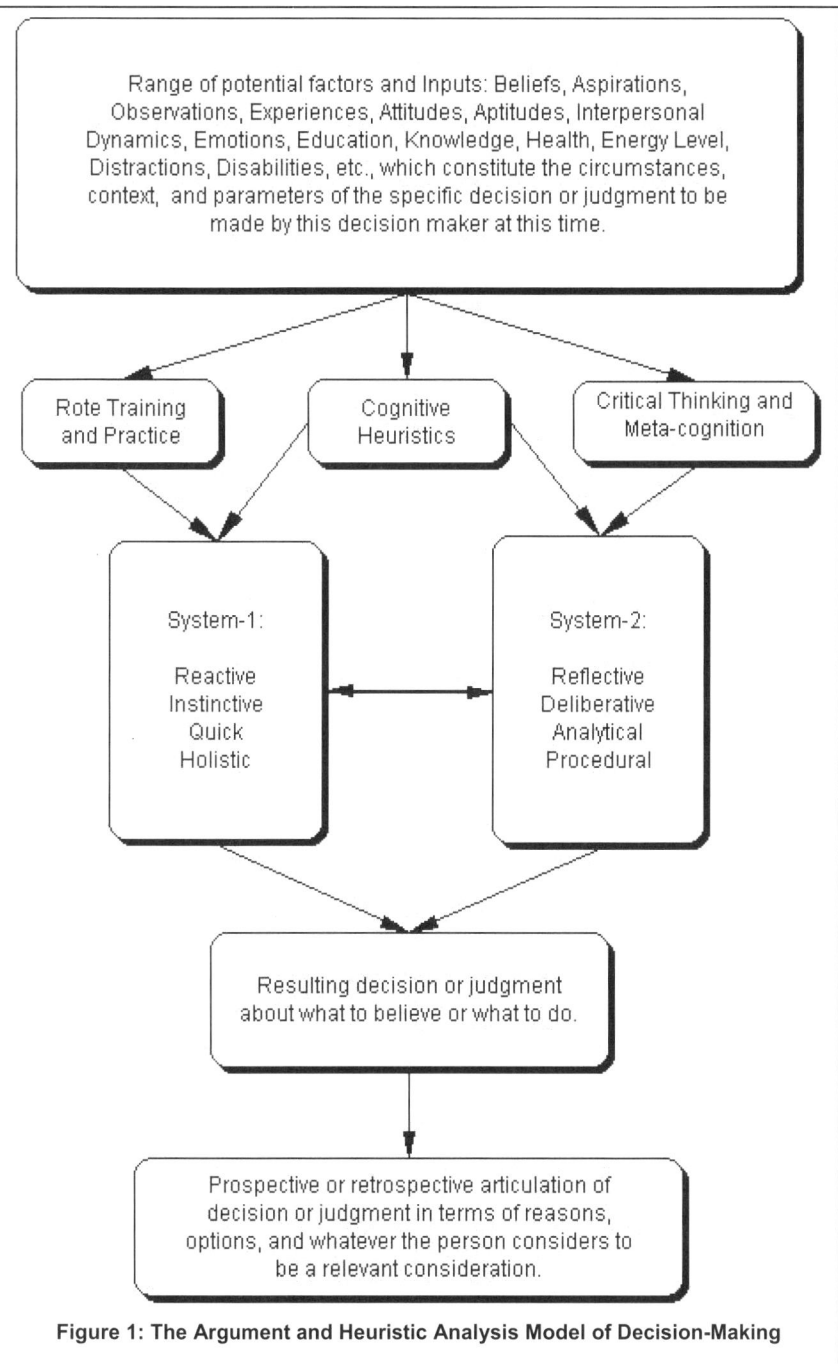

**Figure 1: The Argument and Heuristic Analysis Model of Decision-Making**

mixing System 1 and System 2 cognitive maneuvers to identify and resolve clinical problems is the normal form of mental processes involved in sound, expert, clinical reasoning. Misusing heuristic reasoning maneuvers, in the context of poor logic and misinformation is a description of poor clinical reasoning. Figure 1 below is a diagram locating the thinking processes we have been discussing. Even good thinkers make both System 1 and 2 errors from time to time. We misinterpret things, overestimate or underestimate our chances of succeeding, rely on mistaken analogies, reject options out of hand, rely too heavily on feelings and hunches, judge things credible when they are not, etc. And there is one more strategy humans use to become confident about their decisions which needs to be factored in before the story of clinical reasoning is fully told.

**Dominance structuring**

Richly considered judgments about what to believe or do are typically structured around one dominant conclusion. In the case of a clinical judgment made under risky and uncertain conditions, that judgment emerges as a function of eliminating possible choices based on the evidence available. Subsequently, even when new evidence becomes available that changes the value of the chosen alternative, it proves difficult to override one's original conclusion. This remains true, even when new information renders the supporting reasons for the initial decision questionable at best. Creation of a 'dominance structure' (Montgomery, 1989) around one's choice of action (or inaction) can sustain confidence in the judgment even when the negative consequences of error are extremely high.

We all do this. We need to do this, actually, to attain significant confidence to act under uncertain conditions. Otherwise we would be more likely to delay a needed judgment or fail to maintain our resolve, thus making errors of omission. This would constitute a breech in the trust placed in us as health care providers. But there are dangers here. We can all think of situations where an ineffective plan of care was continued too long to be optimal, and was even harmful for a given individual. If we add the realities surrounding the interpersonal power structure necessary for the function of a medical team, there is an added pressure of responsibility on team leaders to be aware of dominance structures around particular diagnostic or treatment decisions which they may be sustaining long past their utility for improving the health of individual patients. The same situation could be described in relationship to the retention of policies and practices well beyond their appropriate application, or negative judgments against co-workers because initial negative impressions are wrongly sustained.

**Problem parameters**

When we interpret presenting symptoms, we explore their characteristics (frequency, severity, persistence, duration...), knowing that these characteristics modify the symptoms' meaning. So it is with the characteristics of clinical problems, or all of life's problems for that matter. A problem's attributes pose differing challenges for the thinking skills and habits of mind required for successful problem resolution. We have already mentioned above that new, or novel, problems and situations are approached differently than familiar ones. Other key characteristics of problem situations are the associated risk, the problem's complexity, the spontaneity of its occurrence, accompanying time constraints, and the need for specialized knowledge or collaboration required to address a response. Reflect on the likely characteristics of the typical problems presented in clinical practice and recall your own initial clinical experiences as a student. When you were a health science student yourself, many of the problems you encountered in the clinical setting appeared to you to be: 1) novel, 2) complex, 3) high stakes, 4) time constrained, 5) spontaneous, and 6) requiring of more specialized knowledge than you had at your fingertips. Finally, in spite of being a trainee, often you probably felt you had to resolve problems individually rather than relying on collaboration. Your responses to those same problems now will depend in part on the nature of your current practice and the expertise you have developed. The perceived risk attached may be similar, as most clinical judgments are high stakes for you as well as your patients. But there are probably a higher proportion of those problems which are now, for you, highly familiar, less complex, more anticipatable, more within your knowledge base, where time to think is less of an issue, and you can rely on collaboration with other members of the health care team.

Training clinical judgment across all of these possible problem parameters requires a careful pedagogical approach. We need to remember to provide time for trainees to think. Scaffolding the complexity of problems presented to students and novice staff will improve their ability to think well. Debriefing case outcomes as to the embedded clinical reasoning (surfacing assumptions, preliminary diagnoses, suspected interacting factors) externalizes the reasoning process so that it can be critiqued or praised. In the end, training health professionals to think well in clinical practice is a delicate dance, balancing the need to function in swiftly evolving real world cases with the need to allow every promising student time to develop their critical thinking skills.

The emphasis here is on 'promising.' One thing we have learned in the course of our work in critical thinking measurement is that many students admitted to health science programs do not have the requisite thinking skills to become great or even competent diagnosticians. We know this by examining thousands of critical thinking test scores from students across the health science disciplines (Facione & Facione, 1997; Chirema, 2006) and from the research that has been done to link critical thinking test scores with success on licensure examinations in the health sciences (Williams, Schmidt, Tilliss *et. al.*, 2006).

Taking a critical thinking approach to clinical practice entails two linked goals: accurate problem identification and optimal problem resolution. The first is essential. Taking action to solve the wrong problem may work occasionally in politics, but will not work for the sick and dying. The second is also essential. What are the consequences of not taking a critical thinking approach to developing a clinical treatment plan? If clinicians or our health science students do not have the possibility to think reflectively about clinical situations, they will use other methods for problem resolution. Some alternatives to critical thinking are: 1) to ask someone else what to do; 2) to do nothing; 3) to keep on doing something which is failing to achieve our desired outcome; or 4) to do something, anything, new just because it has not been tried yet. The first three are a recipe for mediocrity or failure through omission. The fourth is perhaps most dangerous if the presumed diagnosis is mistaken or if the chanced upon trial treatment turns out to be not simply ineffectual but actually harmful.

At its best, a focus on reflective thinking, and some attempt to meta-cognitively monitor our use of heuristic thinking, allows one to be thoughtful about intellectual honesty, analytically anticipating what happens next, demanding the wisdom of making decisions in a fair-minded and timely manner, and the attempt to eliminate personal biases. These habits of mind have been identified as those of the ideal critical thinker (Facione, Facione & Sanchez, 1994; American Philosophical Association, 1990).

**Multiple measurement modalities**

The assessment of critical thinking lends itself to the full array of measurement methods. Here as in all areas of measurement, multiple measures allow the assessment of critical thinking in the many clinical practice contexts. Multiple choice (Facione & Facione, 2006; Facione, 2000; Watson & Glaser, 1980; Ennis, Millman & Tomko, 1985) or short answer essay tests (Ennis & Weir, 1985), can be used to take one measure of critical thinking skill. These are particularly useful as diagnostic tests for reasoning competence for newly hired clinicians, health science students, and even health care clients who are not cognitively impaired. Some of these instruments use multiple choice questions requiring test-takers to apply critical thinking skills not only to solve a problem but to evaluate the quality of the solution and provide the evidence for that quality. Likert-style attitudinal measures can gauge critical thinking habits of mind (Facione & Facione 1992; Giancarlo 1998). Others have reported the utility of the multiple choice format to test reasoning process when the items are written well (Leung, Mok & Wong, 2007). Rubrics can be constructed to assess particular critical thinking skills or to obtain a holistic ratings of critical thinking skills and disposition. When care is taken to train rater and assure their valid and reliable observation of critical thinking as it presents in real time, these rubrics can be used to assess critical thinking exhibited by clinicians or students in routine case conferences, planned classroom presentations, written assignments, or immediately after addressing a spontaneous bedside situation (Facione & Facione 1996b; Facione & Facione, 1994).

Each assessment device has different potential for assessing critical thinking in relation to more or less authentic clinical judgment situations. Any test of critical thinking must call forth evidence of critical thinking itself and not merely evidence of content knowledge if they are to assess an individual's ability to think well. Psychological measures of critical thinking disposition can provide a barometer for whether a given individual is disposed to use their critical thinking skills rather than to rely on some other way of dealing with problems. These test an individual's willingness to try to think well. We need clinicians who are both willing and able to think well.

**Summary**

The focus on the need to training clinical judgment per se is rather new. At every level from novice to expert, clinical judgment regarding diagnosis, treatment, and on-going evaluation of patient outcomes is a fundamentally complex reasoning process which is applied to problems characterized by a multiplicity of potentially varying parameters, and which consumes cognitive resources including time to think as it relies upon core critical thinking skills and habits of mind, integrating our two systems of decision-making, susceptible to the benefits and shortcomings of cognitive dominance structuring. How clinical reasoning is experience, even d by the expert, is not a reliable measure of either the complexity or the quality of reasoning process. We would make an analogy to the practiced use of customized software on a computer. The apparent ease of the experience belies the cognitive, physiological and mechanical processes at work. We cannot make this point strongly enough, because the potential implications of overconfidence in one's expertise in clinical reasoning could not be more grave for the sick and dying. Previously we were overly confident that students and novice clinicians would somehow "naturally" advance in their clinical reasoning as they were introduced to typical clinical case scenarios. But we have learned that without a direct focus on the critical thinking processes used to interpret, analyze, infer, evaluate, and explain what is going on, progress in clinical reasoning is an uncertain outcome. True, this progress may come entirely from the learners own awareness of how she or he needs to go about internalizing and growing their clinical reasoning expertise. But when wise instructors and mentors facilitate reflective problem-solving by prompting meta-analysis and evaluation of clinical reasoning through their course assignments and pedagogical approaches, the progress is more certain. Changes in health science curricula to case-based pedagogies and problem based learning are relatively recent, but we are already seeing evidence of improved outcomes as educational researchers report that their pedagogical efforts to improve clinical reasoning skills and dispositions have been demonstrated in a variety of health science disciplines and contexts (Jenicek 2006; McAllister 2005; Tiwari, Lai, So & Yuen, 2006, Shin, Jung, Shin, & Kim, 2006; Torre, Daley, Stark-Schweitzer, Siddhartha, et al., 2007; Ozturk, Muslu & Dicle, 2007; Suliman, 2006; Velde & Wittman, 2006). Expanding our knowledge of how to do this well will surely follow.

## References

Ackerman, M., Rinchuse D. & Rinchuse D. (2006). ABO certification in the age of evidence and enhancement. *American Journal of Orthodontics, Dentofacial, and Orthotics*. Vol. 130 (2), 133-140.

American Philosophical Association [APA] (1990). *Critical Thinking: A Statement of Expert Consensus for Purposes of Educational Assessment and Instruction, Recommendations Prepared for the Committee on Pre-College Philosophy*. ERIC Doc. No. ED 315-423.

Benner, P. *From Novice to Expert: Excellence and Power in Clinical Practice*. Menlo Park, CA: Addison Wesley., 1984.

Benner, P. (2004). Using the Dreyfus Model of Skill Acquisition to Describe and Interpret Skill Acquisition and Clinical Judgment in Nursing Practice and Education, *Bulletin of Science, Technology & Society*, Vol. 24, No. 3, 188-199.

Chirema, K. (2006). The use of reflective journals in the promotion of reflection and learning in post-registration nursing students. *Nursing Education Today*, 27,192-202.

Ennis, R. Millman, J. & Tomko, T. *The Cornell CT Test (Levels X and Z)*. Pacific Grove, CA: Midwest Publications, 1985.

Ennis, R & Weir, E. *The Ennis-Weir CT Essay Test: An Instrument for Testing and Teaching*. Pacific Grove, CA: Midwest Publications, 1985.

Facione, N. & Facione, P. (1996a). Externalizing the critical thinking in knowledge development and clinical judgment. *Nursing Outlook*, 44, 129-136.

Facione, N. & Facione P. *Critical Thinking Assessment in Nursing Education Programs: An Aggregate Data Analysis*. Millbrae, CA: California Academic Press, 1997.

Facione, N. & Facione, P. (2006) The cognitive structuring of patient delay. *Social Science & Medicine*, Vol. 63, pp. 3137-3149.

Facione, N. & Facione P. *The Health Sciences Reasoning Test (HSRT)*. Millbrae, CA: California Academic Press, 2006.

Facione, N, Facione, P & Sanchez, C. (1994). Critical thinking disposition as a measure of competent clinical judgment: The development of the California Critical Thinking Disposition Inventory. *Journal of Nursing Education*, 33 (8), 345-350.

Facione, P. *The California Critical Thinking Skills Test (CCTST)*. Millbrae, CA: California Academic Press, 2000.

Facione, P. & Facione, N. *The California Critical Thinking Disposition Inventory (CCTDI)*. Millbrae, CA: California Academic Press, 1992.

Facione, P. & Facione, N. *The Professional Judgment Rating Form: Novice/Intern Level*. Millbrae, CA: California Academic Press, 1996b.

Facione, P. & Facione, N. *Thinking and Reasoning in Human Decision Making: The Method of Argument and Heuristic Analysis*. Millbrae, CA: The California Academic Press, 2007.

Facione, P, Facione, N, & Giancarlo, C, (2000). The Disposition toward critical thinking: Its character, measurement, and relationship to critical thinking skill. *Informal Logic,* Vol. 20 (1), 61-84.

Giancarlo, C, (1998). *The California Measure of Mental Motivation (CM3)*. Millbrae, CA: California Academic Press. 1998.

Gilovic T, Griffin D, & Kahneman D, *Heuristics and biases: The psychology of intuitive judgment.* Cambridge, UK: Cambridge University Press, 2002.

Jenicek, M. (2006). How to read, understand, and write 'Discussion' sections in medical articles. An exercise in critical thinking. *Medical Science Monitor.* 12(6): SR28-36. Epub 2006, May 29.

Jones, B. & Ratcliff, J. National Center on Post Secondary Teaching, (1993). Learning and Assessment, The Pennsylvania State University. US Department of Education's Office of Educational Research and Improvement (OERI) Grant No.: R117610037, CFDA No.:84.117G.

Kahneman, D. Slovic, P. & Tversky, A. *Judgment under Uncertainty: Heuristics and Biases.* Cambridge, UK: Cambridge University Press, 1982.

Leung, S.F., Mok, E. & Wong, D. (2007). The impact of assessment methods on the learning of nursing students. *Nursing Education Today*, Epub ahead of print at the time of this printing.

McAllister, M. (2005). Transformative teaching in nursing education: leading by example. *Collegian*, Vol. 12 (2), 11-6.

Montgomery, H. From cognition to action: The search for dominance in decision making. In, *Process and Structure in Human Decision-Making*, (pp 23-49). John Wiley & Sons Chichester, UK, 1989.

Newell, A. *Toward Unified Theories of Cognition*. Cambridge, MA. Harvard University Press, 1990.

Ozturk, C., Muslu, G.K., Dicle, A. (2007, Dec 1). A comparison of problem based and traditional education on nursing students' critical thinking dispositions. *Nursing Education Today* (epub ahead of print at this printing).

Shin, K, Jung, D, Shin, S, & Kim, M. (2006). Critical thinking dispositions and skills of senior nursing students in associate, baccalaureate, and RN to BSN programs. *Journal of Nursing Education*, Vol. 45 (6), 233-7.

Suliman, W. (2006). Critical thinking and learning styles of students in conventional and accelerated programs. *International Nursing Review*, Vol. 53, 73-79.

Tiwari, A., Lai, P. So, M., & Yuen, F. (2006). A comparison of the effects of problem-based learning and lecturing on the development of students' critical thinking, *Medical Education*, 40, 547-554.

Torre, DM., Daley, B., Stark-Schweitzer, T., Siddhartha, S., Petkova, J., & Ziebert, M. (2007). A qualitative evaluation of Medical student learning with concept mapping. *Medical Teaching*, 29(9), 949-955.

Tversky, A. & Kahneman D, (1973). Availability: A Heuristic for Judging Frequency and Probability. *Cognitive Psychology.* Vol. 5: pp. 207-232.

Velde, B. Wittman, P. & Vos, P. (2006). Development of critical thinking in occupational therapy students. *Occupational Therapy International*. Vol. 13 (1), 49-60.

Watson, G. & Glaser, E. *Watson-Glaser Critical Thinking Appraisal, Forms A and B*. New York: Psychological Corporation, 1980.

Weinstein, N. (1982). Unrealistic optimism about susceptibility to health problems. *Journal of Behavioral Medicine*. Vol. 5. pp. 441-460.

Williams, K, Schmidt, C, Tilliss, T, Wilkins, K, & Glasnapp, D. (2006). Predictive validity of critical thinking skills and disposition for the national board dental hygiene examination: a preliminary investigation. *Journal of Dental Education*. 70(5), 536-44.

# Interpreting Benevolence and Righteousness in Contemporary Health Care

## *Agnes Tiwari & K. H. Yuen*

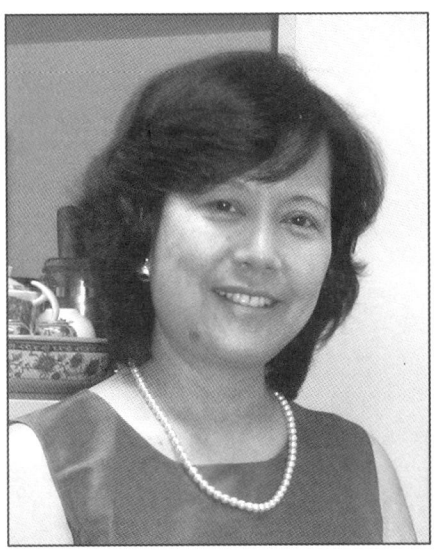

*Dr. Agnes Tiwari is an associate professor in the Department of Nursing Studies, at The University of Hong Kong. Dr. K. H. (Felix) Yuen is a Teaching Consultant, Department of Nursing Studies, The University of Hong Kong. Together they have collaborated on a number of studies of the effectiveness of varying teaching strategies to strengthen critical thinking disposition. Their paper showing the continuing positive effects of Problem-Based Learning on CT dispositions was published in 2006 in Medical Education. (The reference and an abstract are included at the end of this chapter.)*

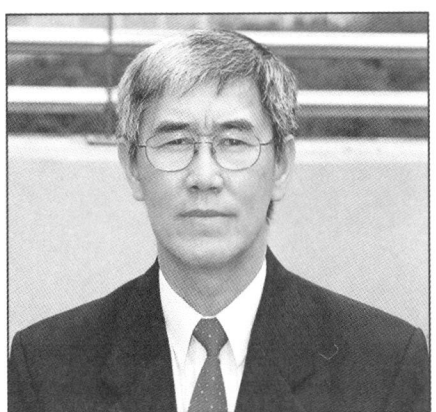

*With Hong Kong now seeking to identify the essential learning outcomes of its educational programs, Dr. Tiwari and her research team are assisting by delineating more fully the manifestations of good critical thinking and clinical judgment in professional practice. We are as eager to see the fruits of this work as we were years ago when she and her team achieved a culturally competent authorized Chinese translation of the California Critical Thinking Disposition Inventory (CCTDI) for use in Hong Kong.*

*In this chapter Tiwari and Yuen bring us a thoughtful discussion of the impact of culture on the expression of thinking and judgment. The context of the lesson is health care ethics built on a traditional reading about the ethical assumptions behind everyday discourse. Finally, this lesson includes a well integrated assessment of progress in developing critical thinking skills. This assessment is done by the professors, and, perhaps just as importantly, it is performed by the students themselves. This type of internalization of the criteria for demonstrating strength does much for developing the habits of mind of demanding strong critical thinking dispositions. This chapter is a jewel of a lesson – one to be contemplated and remembered.*

## Class session and students

This is an example taken from a class we teach to the master of nursing students. The class is the first session in the Philosophy & Science of Nursing course. As is true of most students in Hong Kong, our nursing students come from a Chinese culture with a highly competitive, examination-oriented, and teacher-dominated educational experience. Although the 'traditional' Chinese culture has been modified in recent decades with increasing contacts with the Western culture, some elements of the tradition remain, particularly in aspects of childrearing and education. An emphasis on social harmony and affective control would be the norm for our students while challenging authoritative statements and expressing their private thoughts publicly would not come naturally to them. Furthermore, they would expect classroom activities to be a means of acquiring words of wisdom from the knowledgeable teachers/professors rather than a forum for them to engage in dialectical discussion. One of the objectives of the Philosophy & Science of Nursing course is therefore to encourage students to break free from an authoritarian tradition that has inhibited their desire to search for meaning and truth.

## The goal of the class session

Our goal in this class for our students is that they should strengthen their critical thinking skills and be better able to integrate the skills with confidence and good judgment in their professional work. We mainly focus on the skills of interpretation, analysis, evaluation and explanation as these are more likely to be under-developed in our students given their educational experience in a teacher-dominated, hierarchical and didactic classroom.

## The actual material used for the class session

We have purposefully selected a short chapter on the principles of benevolence and righteousness taken from the Book of Mencius (Table 1), an authoritative seminal work that would not be unfamiliar to our students. *Challenging authoritative statements, however, would be a novel undertaking for the students* as the usual way of learning such seminal work is by understanding the teaching of the master (Mencius in this case) and adopting the authoritative principles in their daily practice. By asking the students to conduct a critical appraisal of Mencius' teaching on benevolence and righteousness and to provide justifications for their conclusion, we seek to promote their skills in interpreting statements, analyzing arguments, assessing claims and presenting reasoning. With practice, we hope that the students would acquire confidence in and develop an inclination to applying their critical thinking skills to authentic life or work situations.

## Learning objectives

By examining the Chapter on Benevolence and Righteousness taken from the Book of Mencius, students who participate in this lesson will be able to:

1) comprehend and express the meaning of benevolence and righteousness in the contemporary healthcare context;

2) identify the reasons in support of their opinions regarding the importance of applying the principles of benevolence and righteousness to the provision of healthcare;

3) assess the credibility of their expressed opinions; and

4) justify their reasoning in terms of evidential or conceptual considerations.

## What we do before class even begins

Before the class, we need to prepare the material for the discussion, which includes the original Chinese version of the Chapter on Benevolence and Righteousness and its English translation (Table 1). The English translation is necessary because many of the students would have some difficulty reading the writing of Mencius as it is not written in modern Chinese. Since the students are adept at reading Chinese and English, a bi-lingual presentation of the Chapter will help them decipher the writing in a less time-consuming manner. We also prepare guidelines to help the students conduct a critical, interactive and hopefully, dialectical discussion. The guidelines are written as a series of critical thinking questions based on the learning objectives of the session (Table 2). We deliberately label the questions as "critical thinking questions" so as to remind the students that they are practicing their skills in critical thinking. Since "critical thinking" is frequently talked about by students and teachers in our tertiary education institutions, it is often treated as a cliché with little regard given to how it is to be acquired or practiced.

**How we teach this lesson**

We start the lesson by reiterating the key thinking that underpins the Philosophy & Science of Nursing course: the advancement of nursing science requires its practitioners to have the skills and inclination to reflect on the quality of one's thinking and to use one's critical thinking skills to engage in more thoughtful thinking and problem-solving in work situations. We tell the students that the Chapter on Benevolence and Righteousness by Mencius provides the context for sharing of views and engagement in mutual and reciprocal critique in this lesson. We then ask the students to read through the Chapter on their own, allowing five minutes or so for this quiet reading activity. More time may be added if necessary. We encourage the students to do their own reading first before moving onto group discussion so that they have a chance to think on their own rather than relying on others' points of view.

After the individual reading, students form discussion groups. Each group consists of 8 - 9 students. Within each group, students further divide into A and B groups for the purpose of completing the group tasks. Table 2 shows the guidelines for group discussion which list the learning objectives and the critical thinking questions for each of the objectives. We choose a seminar room (with capacity for 50 students) for this activity. The groups work through the learning objectives one by one, tackling the critical thinking questions as required. We deliberately give the groups only five minutes to work on each of the objectives as in authentic work situations nurses usually have little time to think before having to respond to problems. Acting as facilitators during the student-led discussion, we assist the groups to focus on the set tasks and adhere to the time allowed for each objective where necessary.

The group's performance during the discussion is observed and recorded unobtrusively using the *Holistic Critical Thinking Scoring Rubric* (HCTSR)[*]. In the first lesson of the course, one of us performs the task of recording these observations, as none of the students would have any experience of using the HCTSR. In the subsequent lessons, two students from each group independently rate the group's performance using the HCTSR. Students rotate to serve as raters so that by the end of the course, every student would have had at least one chance of rating his/her group.

---

[*] The *HCTST*, Facione & Facione, 1994 is reprinted with instructions for use in the final chapter of this teaching anthology.

After the group discussion, a "think-aloud" method is used to provide feedback on the group discussion. In the first lesson, the "think-aloud" is led by the facilitator. With reference to the different levels of the HCTSR, a description of the group's performance while tackling the critical thinking questions during group discussion is read out. Where possible, verbatim transcripts of the discussion are used to illustrate the level of the HCTSR demonstrated by the group. For example, in the first lesson, biased interpretation of evidence is detected in the group discussion in which a group member declares that the local private hospitals are only concerned about "*li*" (financial gains) and only the public hospitals can afford to care about benevolence and righteousness in health care provisions. The member's interpretation reflects her biased assumption that private patients have to pay a large sum for their care whereas patients in public hospitals have only to pay a nominal amount. In reality, her assumption is not upheld as competition among private hospitals has helped to ensure that private care is affordable for a greater number of health care users while health budget cuts have necessitated public hospitals to impose charges at a market price for a number of diagnostic procedures and operations. The group does not question her biased interpretation. In the ensuing discussion, it soon becomes apparent that the group has failed to question the meaning of Mencius' principles of benevolence and righteousness. By highlighting the deficits based on the HCTSR, we are then able to work with the group members in improving their critical thinking skills.

While facilitator-led "think-aloud" is useful in providing feedback, peer-led "think-aloud" is more beneficial for group learning in terms of enhancing critical thinking skills. Therefore, we use facilitator-led "think-aloud" for the first lesson only and peer-led "think-aloud" is conducted for the rest of the course. The role of the facilitators during peer-led "think-aloud" is to act as critical peers, which includes questioning assumptions or demanding justifications where appropriate.

**Feedback from the students**

Initially, students may not be used to this format of learning. They may be confused about their role in the group discussion, for example, those in Group A may perform the tasks assigned to Group B if the latter fails to perform well, and vice versa. Discussion, at the early stage, tends to be superficial and descriptive, with little evidence of dialectical debate. Assumptions are often offered and accepted with little questioning. After the facilitator-led "think-aloud", most of the students would realise where they need to improve. But the most noticeable improvement comes when students take charge of their own rating of performance and "think-aloud". This is particularly true for the raters who have to give feedback to group members.

Subsequent to their experience in providing the "think-aloud", the student-raters generally take a more critical stance and provide a more noticeable leadership in the ensuing group discussions. The impact of the "think-aloud" is best illustrated by the student who demonstrated a biased interpretation as described earlier. At the end of the first lesson, she approached one of the authors and expressed her difficulty to hold her own view when facing people with authority. She was helped to analyze her own deficits in critical thinking and work out some remedial measures. After several rounds of "think-aloud", not only was she playing a more active role in the group discussion, she was evidently more thoughtful when analyzing points of view and more confident in justifying her decisions. Her group's performance also improved from level 2 (at the first lesson) to level 4 (at the sixth lesson) of the HCTSR.

**Table 1. Benevolence and righteousness from the Book of Mencius**

梁惠王章句上．第一章

孟子見梁惠王。

王曰，"叟，不遠千里而來，亦將有以利吾國乎？"

孟子對曰，"王何必曰利？亦有仁義而已矣。"

"王曰：『何以利吾國？』大夫曰：『何以利吾家？』
士庶人曰：『何以利吾身？』上下交征利，而國危矣！
萬乘之國弒其君者，必千乘之家；千乘之國，弒其君者，必百乘之家。
萬取千焉，千取百焉，不為不多矣；□為後義而先利，不奪不饜。"

"未有仁而遺其親者也，未有義而後其君者也。"

"王亦曰仁義而已矣，何必曰利？"

> **The Works of Mencius**
>
> **Book 1, Part I: King Hûi of Liang**
>
> **Chapter I.** *Benevolence and righteousness*
>
> *Mencius's only topics with the princes of his time; and the only principles which can make a country prosperous.*
>
> 1. Mencius went to see king Hûi of Liang.
>
> 2. The king said, 'Venerable sir, since you have not counted it far to come here, a distance of a thousand lî, may I presume that you are provided with counsels to profit my kingdom?'
>
> 3. Mencius replied, 'Why must your Majesty use that word "profit?" What I am provided with are counsels to benevolence and righteousness, and these are my only topics.
>
> 4. 'If your Majesty says, "What is to be done to profit my kingdom?" the great officers will say, "What is to be done to profit our families?" and the inferior officers and the common people will say, "What is to be done to profit our persons?" Superiors and inferiors will try to snatch this profit the one from the other, and the kingdom will be endangered. In the kingdom of ten thousand chariots, the murderer of his sovereign shall be the chief of a family of a thousand chariots. In the kingdom of a thousand chariots, the murderer of his prince shall be the chief of a family of a hundred chariots. To have a thousand in ten thousand, and a hundred in a thousand, cannot be said not to be a large allotment, but if righteousness be put last, and profit be put first, they will not be satisfied without snatching all.
>
> 5. 'There never has been a benevolent man who neglected his parents. There never has been a righteous man who made his sovereign an after consideration.
>
> 6. 'Let your Majesty also say, "Benevolence and righteousness, and let these be your only themes." Why must you use that word -- "profit?"

**Figure 1. Benevolence and righteousness from the Book of Mencius**

TABLE 2. GUIDELINES FOR GROUP DISCUSSION: THE APPLICATION OF THE PRINCIPLES OF BENEVOLENCE AND RIGHTEOUSNESS TO THE CONTEMPORARY HEALTHCARE CONTEXT

| | Learning Objectives | Critical Thinking Questions |
|---|---|---|
| 1. | To comprehend and express the meaning of benevolence and righteousness in the contemporary healthcare context | Group A to pose the question: "Should Mencius' principles of benevolence and righteousness, rather than "*lì*" (financial gain), be the guiding principles for providing healthcare?" (May follow up on the answers provided by group B as appropriate) |
| | | Group B to respond to the question and follow-up questions. |
| 2. | To identify the reasons in support of their opinions regarding the importance of applying the principles of benevolence and righteousness to the provision of healthcare | Group A to pose the question: "Why do you think that?" (May further explore the answers provided by group B) |
| | | Group B to respond to the question and follow-up questions. |
| 3. | To assess the credibility of their expressed opinions | Group A to determine if the reasons given by group B are likely to be true or false and may ask group B to provide new information to further confirm their expressed opinion. |
| | | Group B to respond to group A's request for further confirmation as necessary. |
| 4. | To justify their reasoning in terms of evidential or conceptual considerations | Group B to justify the reasoning upon which their position on the importance of applying the principles of benevolence and righteousness to the provision of healthcare is based: "we believe that benevolence and righteousness are/are not important guiding principles in the provision of healthcare based on the following evidence and counter-evidence…" |
| | | Group A to express their approval or disapproval of group B's justifications. |

## Reference

"A comparison of the effects of problem-based learning and lecturing on the development of students' critical thinking," Authors: Tiwari, Agnes; Lai, Patrick; So, Mike; Yuen, Kwan. Source: Medical Education, Volume 40, Number 6, June 2006, pp. 547-554(8). Publisher: Blackwell Publishing.

*Abstract:* Educational approaches are thought to have facilitative or hindering effects on students' critical thinking development. The aim of this study was to compare the effects of problem-based learning (PBL) and lecturing approaches on the development of students' critical thinking. Method -- All 79 Year 1 undergraduate nursing students at a university in Hong Kong were randomly assigned to 1 of 2 parallel courses delivered by either PBL (n=40) or lecturing (n=39) over 1 academic year. The primary outcome measure was students' critical thinking disposition as measured by the California Critical Thinking Disposition Inventory (CCTDI). Individual interviews were also conducted to elicit the students' perceptions of their learning experience. Data were collected at 4 time-points spanning 3 years. Results -- The overall CCTDI and subscale scores for the PBL group were not significantly different from those of the lecture group at the first time-point (pretest). Compared with lecture students, PBL students showed significantly greater improvement in overall CCTDI ($P=0.0048$), Truthseeking ($P=0.0008$), Analyticity ($P=0.0368$) and Critical Thinking Self-confidence ($P=0.0342$) subscale scores from the first to the second time-points; in overall CCTDI ($P=0.0083$), Truthseeking ($P=0.0090$) and Analyticity ($P=0.0354$) subscale scores from the first to the third time-points; and in Truthseeking ($P=0.0173$) and Systematicity ($P=0.0440$) subscale scores from the first to the fourth time-points. Conclusions -- There were significant differences in the development of students' critical thinking dispositions between those who undertook the PBL and lecture courses, respectively.

# Nurturing Students' Meta-Cognition and Self Reflection Through On-line Journaling

## *Carol Giancarlo-Gittens*

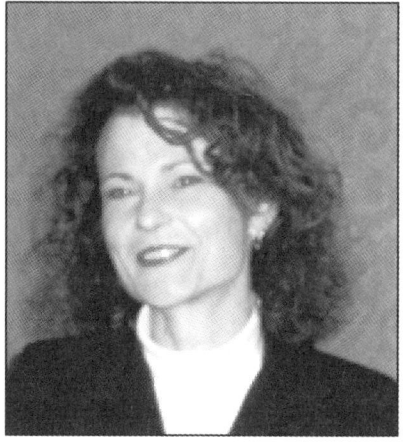

*Dr Carol Giancarlo-Gittens is an Associate Professor of Education and Liberal Studies at Santa Clara University. She serves as the university's Director of Assessment as well as the Associate Dean of the School of Education, Counseling Psychology and Pastoral Ministries. In addition to her administrative roles, Dr. Giancarlo-Gittens teaches critical thinking pedagogy, developmental psychology, foundations of education, curriculum innovation, educational assessment, research methods, and community health education. Her research examines the relationship between critical thinking, motivation, and academic achievement in adolescent and young adult samples. She is author of the California Measure of Mental Motivation (CM3), a critical thinking disposition assessment instrument for children, adolescents and adults, and the Adolescent Reasoning Test (ART) a critical thinking skills test for adolescents. We've included these references at the end of the chapter.*

*In this chapter, Dr. Giancarlo-Gittens describes the use of computer-mediated communication (CMC) to provide students with the opportunity to more deeply interpret, analyze and draw inferences from classroom content or field experiences. The lesson brings important insights not found elsewhere in this volume on how to focus the training of thinking on specific skills(problem framing, analysis of consequences, and the explanation of evaluation). Dr Giancarlo-Gittens presents the Critical Thinking (CT) Reflective Log, an online journaling assignment that was first developed to nurture pre-service teachers' reflective and meta-cognitive skills. It is a wonderfully adaptable lesson for students and clinicians at all levels of practice, well referenced to assist those new to the field of educational research, and it offers a focused effort to build skills in meta-cognitive awareness and critical reflection.*

**Background and Context**

As computer-mediated communication (CMC) becomes more and more common in higher education, learning opportunities expand beyond the physical and temporal boundaries of the university classroom (Frank, 2004; Van Gorp, 1998). Substantial benefits to students result from using CMC to augment face-to-face classroom discussions (Dutt-Doner & Powers, 2000; Frank 2004; Jetton, 2004, MacKnight, 2000; Thomas 2002; Wepner & Mobley, 1998). One of the most noted benefits from using CMC is that it permits students to share and discuss with one another their beliefs and experiences about the content of a course or issues pertaining to field experiences (Andrusyszyn & Davie, 1997; Jetton, 2004; Wepner & Mobley, 1998). A second benefit is that CMC serves as a tool to facilitate collaborations on projects or other shared activities. A third benefit is that CMC provides a virtual learning environment that offers students opportunities to more deeply process information that has been presented in class or is being offered by classmates, and thus to build their critical and reflective thinking skills as they participate in the online discussions (Andrusyszyn & Davie, 1997; Frank, 2004; Harasim, 1990, 2000; Jetton, 2004 Hawkes & Romiszowski, 2001; McComb, 1993, Newman, Johnson, Cochrane & Webb, 1996). The purpose of this paper is to present the Critical Thinking (CT) Reflective Log, an online journaling assignment that was developed with the express purpose of nurturing students' reflective and meta-cognitive skills.

The conceptualization of critical thinking that serves as the foundation for the CT Reflective Log is derived from the consensus definition articulated by the American Philosophical Association (APA). In 1990, under the sponsorship of the APA, a cross-disciplinary panel completed a two-year Delphi project yielding a robust conceptualization of CT understood as an outcome of college level education (Facione, 1990). Before the Delphi Project, no clear consensus definition of critical thinking existed (see Kurfiss, 1988 for a review). Broadly conceived by the Delphi panelists, CT was characterized as the process of purposeful, self-regulatory judgment. Throughout this cognitive, non-linear, recursive process a person gathers and evaluates evidence in order to form a judgment about what to believe or what to do in a given context. In so doing, a person engaged in CT uses his / her cognitive skills to form a judgment and to monitor and improve the quality of that judgment (Facione, 1990).

Contemporary critical thinking scholars acknowledge that any discussion of critical thinking must include both thinking skills and thinking attitudes, or dispositions (Ennis & Norris, 1990; Halpern, 1996). The term critical thinking disposition refers to a person's internal motivation to think critically when faced with problems to solve, ideas to evaluate, or decisions to make (Facione, Facione & Giancarlo, 1997; Giancarlo, Blohm & Urdan, 2004). These attitudes, values, and inclinations are dimensions of one's personality which relate to how likely a person is to approach problem identification and problem solving by using reasoning. Many would agree with the assertion that it is pointless to learn a skill if, when you find yourself in situations that require the skill, you fail to exercise what you have learned. The honing of one's CT skills, as well as developing the disposition to use one's skills, is vital for success in school and throughout a person's life (Halpern, 1998).

Can critical thinking be accomplished in an on-line environment? Astleitner (2002) provides one of the most thorough reviews of the educational literature as to whether critical thinking can be nurtured in an online environment. Astleitner considered multiple modes of electronic communication as well as dynamic differences presented by synchronous versus asynchronous environments. A major contribution stemming from this review was Astleitner's assertion that educators interested in using CMC must craft the online assignment with care, that the assignment be integrated with other course activities, and finally that educators consider the motivational and emotional elements that can impact learning in an online environment (Astleitner, 2002).

Newman and colleagues performed a series of studies to investigate how computer-mediated communication compares to face-to-face interaction in terms of the quality of group learning in college level courses. Newman, Webb and Cochrane (1995), in their examination of students' asynchronous discussion postings, found that students were more likely to provide thoughtful reflection as opposed to novel, creative ideas. They concluded that the asynchronous nature of on-line discussion activities seems best suited for encouraging students to make contemplative, and more considered contributions. The strengths of this line of inquiry include an emphasis on the need to examine the quality of the content of students' on-line discussions not just the quantity or frequency of those interactions (Newman, Webb & Cochrane, 1995).

Issues of democracy, community, gendered discourse and critical thinking within computer-mediated discussions have been investigated. Fauske and Wade (2004) examined whether gendered power differences often seen in face-to-face discussions would also be present in an online discussion assignment in a teacher education course. The authors found that males and females were similar in the tendency to create a supportive, intellectually challenging and inquiry based discussion forums. Fauske and Wade offered recommendations that educators critically examine how they plan and participate in CMC assignments and that asynchronous environments be used to allow students to reflect on their posts to increase the likelihood of thoughtful responses.

## An Overview of the Exercise

This chapter presents a reflective log assignment developed to nurture students' critical and reflective thinking skills. The CT Reflective Log was first created in collaboration with Dr. Peter Facione as an assignment in a senior Capstone seminar for students majoring in Liberal Studies. With experience I've learned that there is more potential benefit to students' critical thinking *if the exercise is introduced early in an educational program.* I further revised this lesson in 2001 when I began *using it with an on-line asynchronous bulletin-board software program to deliver the assignment* as an accompaniment to students' out of class discussion. Well-designed online discussions have been shown to enhance students' inquiry and reflection during field experiences (Dutt-Doner & Powers, 2000; Edens, 2000; Frank, 2004; Wepner & Mobley, 1998).

The CT Reflective Log can be viewed as a form of case study analysis where the students create their own authentic critical thinking case studies based on real life experiences rather than contrived cases created by the professor. Students document the cases and then engage in critical evaluation, analysis and reflection to promote their awareness of strong and weak reasoning as exhibited by others and themselves (Chong, 1998; Jetton, 2004; MacKnight, 2000). The CT Reflective Log is one part of a multifaceted instructional approach that includes a dialogical style of classroom teaching as well as readings that address CT and other topics pertaining to education and the profession of teaching.

## The Learning Outcomes

Students who complete this capstone seminar will be able to:
1. Demonstrate increased meta-cognitive awareness about the role of critical thinking in teaching and learning
2. Infuse one's teaching practices with a pedagogical eye toward critical thinking.
3. Exercise cognitive skills in critical thinking (analysis, inference, interpretation, explanation, evaluation, and meta-cognitive self-regulation).
4. Develop a stronger disposition toward critical thinking (truth-seeking, open-mindedness, analyticity, systematicity, confidence in one's thinking, cognitive maturity).
5. Detect, evaluate, and log striking examples of good and bad thinking in daily life.
6. Demonstrate one's ability to critically evaluate information available (from the Internet and other sources) and develop basic information technological skills.
7. Estimated one's own level of fair-mindedness and critical thinking skill.

## Implementation of the CT Reflective Log

On the first day of class, students receive the CT Reflective Log assignment as part of their course syllabus. I've included the CT Reflective portion here at the end of this chapter so you can refer to it as needed. To complete their assignment, students are asked to integrate a specific new question into their daily conversations each week. The instructor implicitly directs the development of critical thinking through these intentionally crafted weekly questions and the targets of the inquiry specifically identified (King, 1995; MacKnight, 2000). Though students are asked to engage each week with a unique critical thinking reflection prompt, these prompts can be clustered into three major categories: 1) *evaluation of evidence, 2) analysis of alternatives or consequences, and 3) problem identification and problem framing*. Of these, the majority of weekly prompts pertain to the evaluation of evidence. For this first category, prompts from weeks 2, 3, 7 and 9 are relevant. Weekly prompts 4 and 6 serve the second category, and prompts 5 and 8 address the third category. Finally, the last prompt in the assignment requires each student to reflect meta-cognitively on what she or he has learned about his or her own thinking as a result of the journaling activity.

I teach at a university that is on the quarter system and thus there are only nine or ten weeks to implement this assignment. Instructors who teach on a semester system can include additional self-referent prompts of this second categorical type to provide students with more opportunities to overcome the challenges that are presented by reflecting on the degree to which sufficient attention has been paid on anticipating consequences and evaluating alternatives in regards to personal decisions.

Each weekly prompt, students are told, can be modified to reflect their personal style of speech, as long as the main gist of the question remains intact. They are also told specifically to whom the question must be addressed. Sometime the questions must be posed to members of a group (e.g., college graduates, or fellow students not enrolled in the present course), and other times the questions are to be posed to a narrower range of acquaintances, such as best friends, or a professor of their choosing. Finally, some of the questions are reserved for personal reflection. Directing the questions to different targets helps students to generalize their growth in meta-cognition to broader contexts.

## What is expected from class participants?

Each week students are asked to select a salient interaction and post a discussion of that interaction on the class's electronic bulletin board. The description, they are told, should protect the anonymity of those involved, but should provide enough contextual information for the reader to be reasonably able to envision the exchange. I ask my students to first convey the interaction and then evaluate the quality of thinking expressed in the interaction. They are to indicate whether the thinking was strong or weak, and explain why they are making their determination. As an additional layer of complexity to this aspect of the reflective log assignment, out of the nine total posts students will be making throughout the term, only three can be posts recounting encounters deemed to be examples of strong thinking. *The requirement that students must write about examples of weak thinking is based on the idea that, regrettable as it may seem, the most fruitful learning experiences are often negative ones.* Consequently, students are encouraged to strive to find experiences of weak, poor, flawed, fallacious, uncritical, or erroneous thinking. However, since it takes some familiarity with quality to appreciate and to seek excellence in one's own thinking, some of the entries in the log were to be about strong, correct, high quality experiences.

In addition to their original weekly postings, students are obligated to "reply" to at least two other students' posts each week. Early iterations of this assignment asked students to submit their reflections in a handwritten "lab book". As educational technology became more commonplace, the written journals were transitioned to responses emailed to the instructor, and then finally to online bulletin board posts to all in the course. *Along with the transition to a more public submission of the reflections was the addition of online peer replies.* This aspect of the assignment was added as a means for training students' skills in providing professional peer feedback and to lessen the burden on the professor as the sole source of feedback.

**An Analysis of the Design of the Reflective Log Assignment**

Recall that three category areas are covered in the CT Reflective Log: evaluation of evidence (EE), consideration of alternatives and / or consequences (AC) and problem framing (PF). The first question that was considered addressed whether there were any prominent themes stemming from the three categorical prompt types.

***EE: The Evaluation of Evidence.*** Four of the nine prompts ask students to evaluate the extent to which sufficient evidence was being provided to support an asserted claim or point of view. In three of the Evaluation of Evidence prompts the students are asked to solicit and evaluate supporting evidence from another person, and the fourth EE prompt was to evaluate the evidence provided in a television commercial. The goal of the first prompt ("Why do you think that?") is to engage the students in the activity of analyzing the quality of explanation. This explanation provides both a snapshot of the critical thinking skills of the targeted respondent, as well as the skills of the student who must then evaluate the ability to distinguish between *evidence* and *opinion*. The subsequent posts relating to the evaluation of evidence, in weeks 3, 7 and 9 provide students with additional practice in this valuable critical thinking skill, namely the ability to judge the soundness of an argument based on the evaluation of evidentiary support.

**AC: Analysis of Alternatives / Consequences**: Weekly prompts 4 and 6 focus students' attention on the consideration and analysis of alternatives or consequences in a decision-making situation. In the Week 4 prompt, the students are to ask someone who has attained a higher level of education than themselves (in this case a college graduate) 'what else they had considered.' Week 6 asks students to consider the implications of a personal decision. The cognitive skills and dispositions nurtured by these prompts are multifaceted, and differ from the Evaluation of Evidence prompts. When asking a respondent to reflect upon a prior decision, students are exposed to the extent to which the respondent endeavored to identify her or his options, and the degree to which these options were seriously considered. A reflection upon one's own process of identifying alternatives and considering consequences is what confronts students in week 6. The act of seeking to identify options and alternatives is evidence of one's inquisitiveness and open-mindedness. In order to have consequences to consider, we must first desire to identify our options. Furthermore, beyond the brainstorm activity of listing one's choices in any given decision making context, we must exercise skill in analyzing and evaluating the many alternatives in order to identify the best path to take. One's truth-seeking is displayed in this analysis and evaluation process as well in the extent to which the individual desires the "best" decision rather than the easiest or most expeditious decision or conclusion.

*PF: Problem Framing.* Weeks 5 and 8 present students with prompts designed to elicit from others the factors that determined how they framed a particular problem they were facing or had faced in the past. Week 5 requires students to evaluate the problem framing skills of their best friend, and Week 8 asks students to evaluate the problem framing skills of one of their professors. Problem framing, or in other words, problem identification, is one cognitive skill that is often under-developed. More frequently, instructors present problem-solving situations (essay prompts, lab experiments, out-of-class projects, examinations, etc.) where the parameters of the problem are fairly, if not completely, demarcated in advance. There is a reasonable amount of certainty that comes from this advanced staging, namely increased control of the problem-solving situation and increased certainty that the desired learning outcome will be experienced by the students.

The recent pedagogical trend of utilizing problem-based learning (PBL; Duch, Groh, & Allen, 2001) provides teaching method that encourages students to direct their own learning process while working in collaborative groups to solve real-world problems. PBL is an effective strategy for developing students' thinking skills and motivating them to learn across disciplinary boundaries. *Through PBL students are practiced in the pre-problem solving task of determining the nature of the problem, and the parameters of the problem solving situation in addition to deriving an evidence-based solution.* In a similar vein, the Problem Framing prompts of the Reflective Log activity seek to build students' metacognitive awareness of this critical pre-problem solving skill.

**Role of the Instructor during the CT Reflective Log**

It is optimal that the CT Reflective Log be introduced to students at the beginning of a course or program of study. It is particularly important that students are exposed to the online environment, know how to use the particular web-based bulletin board system being used for the exercise, and are comfortable with the software interface so they will be able to successfully post their reflections and reply to their peers. It is also important that students are able to ask questions about the CT Reflective Log activity. *Depending on cultural background, students sometimes need to hear a clear explanation of the importance of the exercise and the reason why they are being asked to evaluate the thinking represented in their own posts and that of their peers.*

I've found that students may not immediately feel confident in their ability to ask the weekly questions, especially if the task requires the student to be more intentional in their queries (i.e., the student might perhaps need to seek out interactions in order to pose the prompt to particular others). This potential was taken into consideration when the CT Reflective Log was developed. The weekly exercise starts with a question that is relatively easy to incorporate into every day conversations – "Why do you think that?" The first target was similarly identified as a familiar "other" – a fellow student / peer. The weekly prompts gradually increase in challenge over the first few weeks in order to allow students to acclimate to the process. *It has been the experience of this author over the past ten years that by Week 4 students typically become quite engaged and enthusiastic about this exercise.* Frequently, students will display an eagerness and intentionality by actively seeking out multiple opportunities to pose the weekly question to see what quality of thinking responses they will receive from different targets and what reactions they receive from their peer group when they make their online posts.

Instructors should thoroughly debrief each week's experiences, but only after students have had an opportunity to post their reflections and reply to their peers. It will be tempting for the instructor who is monitoring the online bulletin board to want to contribute to the discussion. Frank (2004) however suggests that instructors should resist joining as a regular participant in CMC discussions when student-centered learning is the primary goal. The peer group is intended to serve as the source of corrective feedback when a class member's post regarding his or her evaluation of the quality of the target's thinking is inaccurate or insufficiently reflective. *When the instructor is an active and regular participant in the online environment the quality and frequency of thoughtful peer feedback is negatively influenced.* The presence of the knowledgeable authority figure is, in this context, a detriment to peer-supported, student-centered learning.

This is not to say that the instructor must let fallacious thinking and insufficient reflective practice go unnoticed. Instructors may wish to intercede by placing their own post the bulletin board environment. This should be done sparingly and sporadically so as to avoid the anticipation of on-going instructor participation. To facilitate meta-cognitive reflection and the peer feedback process without interacting in the virtual environment, instructors can create a classroom climate that is welcoming of active discussion where self-reflections and peer reactions are encouraged. When necessary, it is in the context of the in-class discussion that the instructor can pose questions to the group that will encourage students to advance their thinking in regards to examples being proffered for a given weekly prompt.

*Thus the primary role of the professor in guiding this activity to nurture critical thinking is to guide the debriefing discussion* by asking students to offer a verbal description of her or his weekly post (the scenario and their evaluation of the quality of the target's reasoning) and to solicit comments from peers in response to the scenario the student is presenting. *It has been my consistent experience that students require guidance in the argument analysis and evaluation process.* In order for this assignment to be optimally effective in nurturing critical thinking, the instructor should use these in class debriefing sessions to discuss techniques of argument evaluation that include a consideration of argument *form* (structure and agreement), *content* (veracity and reliability of claims or conclusions being posited) and *context* (validity and appropriateness of the argument to the situation in which it is being offered).

## Empirical Evaluation of Reflective Logs: Analysis of the Qualitative Data

Using the CT Reflective Log exercise in my classes for the past ten years has generated numerous examples of reflections and peer responses. I've done a qualitative analysis of these reflective examples to observe whether they would reveal a noticeable change in students' critical thinking and reflective practice over the ten-week academic term. The following two questions guided my evaluation of this assignment as to whether it *indeed* nurtured students' critical thinking and reflection: 1) what are the prominent features about the posts from each of the categorical prompts types? And 2) Do students' demonstrate reflective practice in their posts or in their approach to this assignment?

As an attempt to answer these questions, I've included here an analysis of one group of students' prompts drawn from students' posts. There were seventeen students in this group. All seventeen gave posts worthy of quoting; only the most salient of which I've included here, along with my interpretation of their progress on the specified learning objectives.

### Prominent features about posts from each of the thematic prompts types

*EE: The Evaluation of Evidence.* As mentioned above, students begin the journaling assignment in Week 2 by posing a question that is often perceived as one that is easy to incorporate into everyday conversation. For example one student wrote "I really tried hard to incorporate this week's question into my conversations. It was good we started with an easy one so people wouldn't be that taken aback."

For the most part, students seemed to recognize the lack of supportive evidence as indicative of weak thinking. One student in her Week 2 reflection wrote, "This was weak thinking in my opinion because the claim that he made lacked any type of evidence". Another said, "She made her decision through speculation and didn't even stop to think about other possibilities. She let her anger and emotions get the best of her." Correlated to this was the recognition of the need to be open-minded when considering all relevant evidence in a situation. This is reflected in the following student's response to the Week 9 prompt: "I think this is weak thinking. To not take other points of view seriously or to consider all the effects a decision can have is not using critical thinking."

However, there were a small number of instances where the students seemed to be forgiving of the fact that the speaker failed to support their position with evidence, and thus were less likely to deem the thinking as weak. This was a common occurrence in instances where the student felt that the speaker's thinking was being "clouded" by emotions. This is evident in the following quote: "with relationships and feelings, I suppose that some things cannot always be explained." Overall, out of the three categories of question prompts in the CT Reflective Log, the evaluation of evidence seemed to be executed with general ease by most of the students.

*AC: Consideration of Alternatives / Consequences.* Though not explicitly determined by the language of the prompt, the question for Week 4 was usually posed in relation to another's career decision making. Interestingly, this question tended to be asked to the student's parent or older sibling rather than an acquaintance or friend. In most cases the students in this sample reflected upon an impending career decision, namely whether to begin a teaching credential program the following year. In other words, it appears that they focus on the implications of a decision that needs to be made. Notice though that the wording of the prompt is not temporally bound. It is worth mentioning that students who complete this assignment in the spring quarter also focus on a career decision, but by the spring the decision has already been made, so they are reflecting on the implications of an already set decision.

The overwhelming consideration in determining thinking to be strong was whether or not the student felt they saw evidence of open-mindedness and thorough consideration of all possible alternatives during the decision making process rather than logical strength. In her response to Week 4, one student wrote, "I think this was good thinking because she did not have her mind set all along but was open to different options until the one that felt right came along." Another said: "He really considered many options and had legit [sic] reasons why he narrowed some down and went with others. I would call this strong thinking because he gave thought to what he had considered before he answered my question. He also had reasons why he did what he did."

Students were more challenged by the task of evaluating their own thinking in terms of their consideration of alternatives and consequences. Responses to Week 6 where students were asked to reflect on the ramifications of a personal decision exhibited some students' tendency to feel that the process of critical thinking is at times daunting, emotionally charged, and even overwhelming when the decision is deemed to be "high stakes" such as a career decision or relationship decision.

*PF: Problem Framing.* The discussion will be limited here to Week 8 as this was clearly the one prompt of the full set of nine that gave students the most challenge. In some cases, the students were unable to perform this action. Other students took advantage of situations where the question was posed to a professor by another individual. Still another student encountered a situation where it was a professor asking the question rhetorically to his class after the group had performed poorly on a quiz. When debriefing in class about students' difficulty with this week's prompts, students reported discomfort in what they felt was their implicit questioning of their instructor's authority and expertise. This enabled the author to have a wonderful discussion of the role of authority and power in influencing human behavior and impacting the decision making process. We discussed the forceful cognitive heuristic, the human tendency, of deferring to or following perceived authoritative others when determining how to feel or how to act in a given situation.

An overall impression that comes from reading students' posts for Week 8 is that they were surprised by the effect their questioning had on the professor's behavior. One student wrote:

> "I thought [my professor's thinking] was strong because my professor gave me numerous reasons. I also believe this to be strong because she sifted through her notes in order to best answer my question and then she also told me her own personal feelings on it. She was also then able to base what she said upon factual information and gave out specific statistics."

Probably the most moving post for Week 8 came from a student who reflected that she was unable to complete the assignment as planned, but nonetheless still recognized the influence she had on her professor. She wrote:

> "For this week's question I chickened out and asked one of my professors the question via e-mail and not in person; but at least it was asked. I e-mailed my political science teacher and asked her what exactly the problem was with giving women paid or longer maternity leave? After a day or so she e-mailed me back ... she said that she sees a "correlation between who makes the policies (heads of business and government tend to be men) and what they prioritize in business decisions." Then, she sent out an e-mail to the class forwarding an article that she found in the paper that day regarding this issue of women's pay in which it said women just don't negotiate for better pay. So, I would like to think my question sparked her to look for more information on this topic and then find the news article. The fact that she looked for more information on the topic makes me think she really thought about my question. Therefore, I would classify her thinking as strong because she gave me valid reasons and she did further investigating into the topic to back up her opinions."

Many students conveyed observations in their posts for Week 8 that the question caused their professor to deviate from the preplanned lecture or discussion topic. In most cases, students were impressed by their professor's level of enthusiasm and knowledge about their discipline. Finally students reported that the conversation in the classroom became considerably more "interesting" after they posed their question and launched the new class discussion focus. Perhaps one explanation for this experience is the fact that professors often omit the process and problem framing that went into something as grand as a disciplinary theorem or as seemingly mundane as the selection of lecture topics for any given class session. Professors rarely expose students to the thinking process that went into class session planning, but rather restrict presentation to the product of that thinking. Though not a direct goal in this assignment, it is evident from at least some of the prompts that students' gained a sense of empowerment from the practice of asking thought provoking questions of their professors.

## Do students' demonstrate reflective practice in this assignment?

The other question guiding this effectiveness investigation focused directly on the issue of validity. The students' prompts were read with an eye for statements that were indicative of students' reflection. Two modes of reflection were identified. First, students gave examples of reflection during or after the posing of the weekly prompt. Sometimes the examples were of active reflection. One student wrote: "I wasn't even thinking about this class when this conversation happened, but as I reflected upon it after, I realized that it was a perfect example of weak thinking". Other times the students supported their decision for labeling another's thinking as weak by stating that there was a lack of reflection. Consider the following quotes: "I think her thinking was weak because she did not take even a second to think about what I had said." Or "I think that it displayed very weak thinking as he said only the most obvious thing and did not really consider it very much."

The other mode of reflection came in the form of statements students gave to indicate that they were engaging in meta-cognitive reflection on the assignment. One student stated: "I didn't really ask her the question at the right time in the conversation, but I think it fit. Next time I will insert the question better." Another, in response to a television commercial said:

> "I think their reasoning is non-existent. I think my refusal to see the commercial as good advertising for their product is good thinking. It would be dumb of me to see [Brand] as a good choice in response to this commercial since they give no reasoning at all."

A final way to evaluate whether the Reflective Log worked to increase students' meta-cognition and reflection was to examine the students' statements on what they learned about their thinking. Insights about the nature of critical thinking and one's personal skills and dispositions were evident in other students' Week

10 posts. Some of the insights on the nature of CT are reflected in the following quotes:

- I think being a good critical thinker is looking at all sides of the story and figuring out what would be the best solution from that point on.

- I've learned that being a good critical thinker does not always mean that I will find the right or wrong answer, but I know it will help me find the best solution. I'm sure there is more room for me to improve on becoming a better critical thinker, but this class has definitely provided a strong foundation for me.

Many students provided an assessment of their own thinking skills. Some students reflected that they did not consider themselves ones who thought well or often, whereas others recognized that they were strong thinkers, and that the assignment enabled them to be more assured in this self-assessment. This is evident in statements such as the following:

- I've come to the conclusion that I need to practice my critical thinking skills more often.

- I feel questioning other peoples [sic] thinking has really made me understand how little thought most people put into what they have to say, and this has in turn made me more aware of, not only what I choose to agree with, but also how thought out my own statements are.

- There have been times I've been trying to stretch my mind to explain certain things or evaluate thinking in this log and felt like my own thinking wasn't strong enough. However, on the flip side, I also noticed myself becoming more reflective. At my placement I was evaluating and judging every action to ensure that it was beneficial to the students. I was surprised to realize that I was constantly in a state of reflection in this case.

- I have realized the importance of critical thinking in the teaching profession. Reflecting is important to understand what went well or what didn't and why this is so.

## Summary Comments to Guide our Future Research on Meta-cognition

What are the reasons for the effectiveness of this CT Reflective Log assignment? I believe that a key element of this assignment that positively stimulates students' reflective practice is the asynchronous nature of the online environment. There is ample evidence that asynchronous CMC allows students to consider without constraint not only the discussion posted by their peers but their thoughts, feelings and reactions to the discussion before posting a reply (Andrusyszyn & Davie, 1997). Furthermore, the professor is able to interject into the asynchronous discussion in order to provide feedback and scaffolding (Angeli, Valanides & Bonk, 2003, Bullen, 1998; McLoughlin & Luca, 2000). Feedback in this assignment comes in the form of the occasional online corrective comment when a student was applying weak thinking or if thinking was absent, as well in class discussion that focus on improving students' thinking as well as praising examples of strong thinking skills or dispositions.

A unique feature of this assignment as a vehicle for nurturing reflective practice is that the content of the prompts are not based on a specific disciplinary subject matter or context, but rather focus on generalizable CT skills and dispositions. While the CT Reflective Log has been used exclusively in the context of the author's pre-service education courses, it is conceivable that this assignment could be modified to be used in other disciplines. Minnich (2003) argues that social communication is central to the development and active participating in critical thought. The CT Reflective Log serves this social communication purpose, particularly because the vast majority of the weekly prompts are directed at others rather than self-reflection. It is also this idea of social communication that is given opportunity in the online CMC environment. While the examples in this chapter have focused thus far exclusively on the content of the original weekly posts of students, the replies to those posts can provide valuable information about the nature and degree of students' reflection and critical thinking that is possible through CMC.

More can be learned by examining the on-going communication that occurs as a result of this type of exercise. What follows is an example of a string of replies to an original post. This is typical of posts and replies throughout the nine week assignment in the author's undergraduate courses.

> Original Post for Week 10: I feel that this class has made me think critically about critical thinking; that is I learned to better evaluate my own thinking and others. In general, many of us are capable of critical thinking, but often times choose not to use these skills. I wonder why that is. Perhaps it's because it's tiring, or we don't really want to because we're scared of the conclusion or answer we may come to. I think that this is one of the most interesting aspects of critical thinking, simply when we choose to use it.
>
> - REPLY #1: I totally agree. I think it will be interesting now that we are more aware of our own critical thinking to be able to see when we use it and when we don't!

- REPLY #2: Sometimes I think that's the hardest part of critical thinking. It's like when you know what's right for you, but you don't do it anyway because you're scared of the effect.

- REPLY #3: I see what you mean about people not using their critical thinking skills, even though they are capable of it. I actually see myself doing that a lot, but I think it's more because I like to keep things as simple as possible, even though that's not the way things usually end up. But imagine how life would be if we always thought critically about everything...

- REPLY #4: I am also really drawn to when people choose to use critical thinking. Can we stimulate this? Can we motivate this in others?

These exchanges give one a sense of the tone that is created, the habits that are nurtured, and the valuing of the assignment at the end of the ten-week term. What is most encouraging is that the replies to this assignment tended not to be based solely on the content of the original post. Instead, as can be seen above, the replies often times go on to give independent evaluations of the critical thinking evidence, suggest reflective and meta-cognitive activity, and as is the case in Reply #4, go on to pose new questions about pedagogy to enhance critical thinking. These dialogues clearly cannot be achieved through a hard copy journal or email journal that is submitted periodically to the instructor. In summary, this assignment works because it supports the students as they create a mutually supportive community of thinkers.

## References

Andrusyszyn, M. & Davie, L. (1997). Facilitating reflection through interactive journal writing in an online graduate course: A qualitative study. *Journal of Distance Education, 12* (1/2), 103-126.

Angeli, C., Valanides, N. & Bonk, C. J. (2003). Communication in a web-based conferencing system: The quality of computer-mediated interactions. *British Journal of Educational Technology, 34*(1), 31-43.

Astleitner, H. (2002). Teaching critical thinking online. *Journal of Instructional Psychology, 29*(2), 53-76.

Bullen, M. (1998). Participation and critical thinking in online university distance education. *Journal of Distance Education* [WWW document]. URL: http://cade.athabascau.ca/vol3.2/bullen.html.

Chong, S. M. Models of asynchronous computer conferencing for collaborative learning in large college classes. In C. J. Bonk & K. S. King (Eds.), *Electronic collaborators: Learner-centered technologies for literacy, apprenticeship, and discourse* (pp. 157-182). Mahwah, NJ: Lawrence Erlbaum., 1998.

Duch, B. J., Groh, S. E. & Allen, D. E. *The problem of problem based learning: A practical "How To" for teaching undergraduate courses in any discipline.* Sterling, VA: Stylus Publishing, 2001.

Dutt-Doner, K. M. & Powers, S. M. (2000). The use of electronic communication to develop alternative avenues for classroom discussion. *Journal of Technology and Teacher Education, 8*(2), 153-172.

Edens, K. M. (2000). Promoting communication, inquiry, and reflection in an early practicum experience via an on-line discussion group. *Action in Teacher Education, 22* (2), 14-23.

Ennis, R. H. & Norris, S. P. Critical thinking assessment: Status, issues, needs. In S. Legg & J. Algina (Eds.), *Cognitive assessment of language and math outcomes: Advances in discourse processes* (Vol. 46, pp. 1-42). Stamford, CT: Abblex. 1990.

Facione (1990). Critical thinking: A statement of expert consensus for purposes of educational assessment and instruction. *The Delphi Report Executive Summary: Research findings and recommendations prepared for the committee on pre-college philosophy.* ERIC Document No. ED 315-423.

Facione, P. A., Facione, N. C. & Giancarlo, C. A. The motivation to think in working and learning. In E. A. Jones (Ed.) *Preparing competent college graduates: Setting new and higher expectations for student learning, New Directions for Higher Education*, Vol. 96 (pp. 67-79). San Francisco: Jossey-Bass, 1997.

Fauske, J. & Wade, S. E. (2004). Research to practice online: Conditions that foster democracy, community and critical thinking in computer-mediated discussions. *Journal of Research on Technology in Education, 36*(2), 137-153.

Frank, A. M. (2004). Integrating computer mediated communication into a pedagogical education course: Increasing opportunity for reflection. *Journal of Computing in Teacher Education, 20*(2), 81-89.

Giancarlo, C. A., Blohm, S. W., & Urdan, T. (2004). Assessing Secondary Students' Disposition toward Critical Thinking: Development of the California Measure of Mental Motivation. *Educational and Psychological Measurement, 64(2),* 347-364.

Giancarlo-Gittens, C. A. Assessing critical thinking dispositions in an era of high-stakes standardized testing. In J. Sobocan & L. Groake (Eds.), *Critical Thinking, Education and Assessment*, London, Ontario, Canada: The University of Western Ontario through the Althouse Press (In Press).

Halpern, D. F. *Thought and knowledge: An introduction to critical thinking* (3$^{rd}$. Ed.). Mahwah, NJ: Lawrence Erlbaum, 1996.

Halpern, D. F. (1998). Teaching critical thinking for transfer across domains: Dispositions, skills, structure training, and metacognitive monitoring. *American Psychologist, 53*(4), 449-455.

Harasim, L. Online education: An environment for collaboration and intellectual amplification. In L. Harasim (Ed.), *Online education: Perspectives on a new environment* (pp. 39-64). New York: Praeger, 1990.

Harasim, L. (2000). Shift happens: Online education as a new paradigm in learning. *Internet and Higher Education, 3*(1-2), 41-61.

Hawkes, M. & Romiszowski, A. (2001). Examining the reflective outcomes of asynchronous computer-mediated communication on in-service teacher development. *Journal of Technology and Teacher Education, 9*(2), 285-308.

Jetton, T. L. (2004). Using computer-mediated discussion to facilitate pre-service teachers' understanding of literacy assessment and instruction. *Journal of Research on Technology in Education, 36*(2), 171-191.

Kurfiss, J. (1998). *Critical thinking: Theory, research, practice and possibilities.* ASHE-ERIC Higher Education Report No. 2. Washington, DC: Association for the Study of Higher Education.

King, A. (1995). Designing the instructional process to enhance critical thinking across the curriculum: Inquiring minds really do want to know: Using questioning to teach critical thinking. *Teaching of Psychology, 22*(1), 13-18.

MacKnight, C. (2000). Teaching critical thinking through online discussions. *Educause Quarterly, 23*(4), 38-41.

McComb, M. (1993). Augmenting a group discussion course with computer-mediated communication in a small college setting. *Interpersonal Computing and Technology: An Electronic Journal for the 21$^{st}$ Century, 1*(3), Retrieved May 20, 2004, from: http://www.helsinki.fi/science/optek/1993/n3/mccomb.txt

McLoughlin, C. & Luca, J. (2000). Cognitive engagement and higher order thinking through computer conferencing: We know why but do we know how? *Teaching and Learning Forum* [WWW Document].
URL: http://cleo.murdoch.edu.au/confs/tlf/tlf2000/mcloughlin.html

Minnich, E. K. (2003). Teaching thinking: Moral and political considerations. *Change*, Sept. / Oct., 19-24.

Newman, D. R., Johnson, C., Cochrane, C., & Webb, B. (1996). An experiment in group learning technology: Evaluating critical thinking in face-to-face and computer-supported seminars. *Interpersonal Computing and Technology, 4*, 57-74.

Newman, D. R., Webb, B., & Cochrane, C. (1995). A content analysis method to measure critical thinking in face-to-face and computer supported group learning. *Interpersonal Computing and Technology, 3*(2), 56-77.

Thomas, M. (2002). Learning within incoherent structures: The space of online discussion forums. *Journal of Computer Assisted Learning, 18*(3), 351-66.

Van Gorp, M. J. (1998). Computer-mediated communication in pre-service teacher education: Surveying research, identifying problems, and considering needs. *Journal of Computing in Teacher Education, 14*(2), 8-14.

Wepner, S. B. & Mobley, M. M. (1998). Reaping new harvests: Collaboration and communication through field experiences. *Action in Teacher Education, 20*(3), 50-61.

# THE REFLECTIVE LOG

**WHY:** This exercise calls for you to write brief descriptions of *interesting experiences* with regard to thinking critically or scientifically. Meta-cognitive self-correction is the key to becoming a better thinker, and it is the reasoning behind this assignment. Rather than mindlessly repeating one's own errors of reasoning, or being misled by the errors of others, one is able, through meta-cognition, to reflect on one's own thinking. By applying critical thinking skills to the products of one's own critical thinking, one is able to analyze, interpret, explain, and evaluate one's thinking by the standards of good reasoning. One can, in fact, use one's own thinking to correct and to improve one's own thinking. This remarkable human mental ability, known as "meta-cognitive self-correction" is the real engine which drives an individual's and a collaborative team's growth in thinking. It is why good thinking can be found in many people, even those who have not had the benefit of formal education. In some cases, its absence, even in those who have received many years of schooling or "scripted training," is why persons fail to grow and mature as thinkers, and why their reasoning, regardless of their status or power, leaves so much to be desired.

**HOW:** The reflective log activity will begin in **WEEK 2 and will continue through WEEK 10**. Each week, students will post their weekly reflection response as a news item on our class electronic Bulletin Board. In preparation for your weekly post, take notice of the thinking demonstrated around you in relation to the weekly "reflection question". You may find it useful to keep a written record in a notebook to facilitate your recollection. The process and progress of your interpretations, analyses, inferences, evaluations, and explanations will be manifest, albeit probably only in sketchy ways, in these preliminary notes. Since this log is about reflecting on thinking, those preliminary notes are valuable markers to you of the progress and development of your ideas. Each week, when your thinking becomes more developed, compose a ***final paragraph*** for that week. The week's final paragraph must include your reflection and evaluation (strong or weak & why?) of the thinking involved in addition to the date and description of event or circumstance. This final paragraph should be added as a post to the Bulletin Board. **In addition**, each student should COMMENT (reply) on at least two (2) classmates' posts each week. We will discuss these "reflection questions of the week," so come prepared!

**WHAT:** Each week's post must relate a striking experience with regard to thinking critically or scientifically. What is striking for you might not be striking for someone else. It is YOUR experience and your reflection on it that this log is intended to record. Regrettable as it may seem, the most fruitful learning experiences are often negative ones. In responding to the question for each week, you should strive to find experiences of weak, poor, flawed, fallacious, uncritical, or erroneous thinking. On the other hand, since it takes some familiarity with quality to appreciate and to seek excellence, some of the entries in the log must also be about strong, correct, high quality experiences that are striking to you because of how good the scientific or critical thinking was. Of the nine weekly entries, <u>no more than three may be about good thinking</u>. **The post for each week should evaluate (with supporting reasoning) the <u>quality</u> of thinking being discussed.**

### Weekly prompts for the Critical Thinking Reflective Log

| | |
|---|---|
| W2: Why do you think that? (EE) | ASK: Another student (or co-worker), not in this course |
| W3: How good is the evidence for that? (EE) | ASK: Anyone who is stating an opinion, not yourself |
| W4: What else did you consider? (AC) | ASK: Someone who has completed college |
| W5: Exactly why do you say that's the problem? (PF) | ASK: Your best friend |
| W6: What does this decision imply? (AC) | ASK: Yourself |
| W7: How sound is the reason they're giving? (EE) | ASK: Yourself, relative to TV commercial |
| W8: What's really the problem here? (PF) | ASK: A professor |
| W9: What evidence would disconfirm our view? (EE) | ASK: Someone who agrees with you |
| W10: What did I learn about my own thinking? | ASK: Yourself |

| | |
|---|---|
| W11*: What are the consequences of making this decision? (AC) | ASK: Yourself, at least once a day |
| W12: What's really the problem here? (PF) | ASK: Your field / practicum supervisor |
| W13: Are we correct in making this decision /policy? (AC) | ASK: Someone who shares with you the responsibility for making a decision |
| W14: What are the options / alternatives? (AC) | ASK: Yourself in relation to an important decision |
| W15: How strong is our thinking up to this point? (EE) | ASK: Others in a group decision-making moment |

*Note.* The thematic type of each weekly prompt is indicated in parentheses. EE refers to Evaluating Evidence, AC refers to Alternatives / Consequences and PF refers to Problem Framing.

---

* Additional suggested prompts to extend this activity for a semester course.

# Developing On-Line Cases for Teaching Critical Thinking and Clinical Reasoning Skills

*Sara Kim, Doug Brock, Tom Gallagher, Peggy Odegard, Carolyn Prouty, Lynne Robins, and Sarah Shannon,*

*This chapter is for all of us who strive to write case scenarios that will be effective for training clinical reasoning. The chapter has been contributed by a wonderful team of health science educators headed by Dr. Sara Kim at the University of Washington in Seattle. They demonstrate exceptional production of course materials on difficult topic matter by using the disclosure of a medical error as the content area for the on-line lesson. We've included descriptions of the health science roles of all who helped develop this lessons as an example of how others might collaborate to achieve high quality course offerings.*

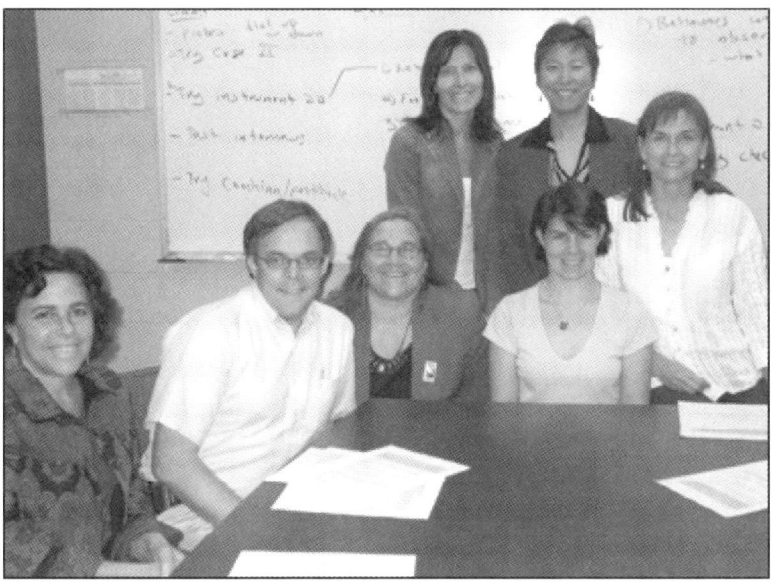

Sitting (from left): Robins, Gallagher, Prouty, Charpentier (Project Coordinator), Shannon. Standing: Odegard, and Kim. Not pictured: Brock

## Bio-sketches of this collaborative team from the University of Washington

***Sara Kim***, Ph.D. is an Associate Professor in the School of Medicine, an adjunct professor in Pediatric Dentistry in the School of Dentistry, and lectures in the College of Education. As the Associate Director of

Education and Curriculum at the Institute for Surgical and Interventional Simulation (ISIS) she oversees the process of developing and peer-reviewing curricular content and Web-based cognitive training tools, and mentors junior faculty members with grant writing and publications. Dr. Kim has implemented and evaluated numerous Web-based distance education tools for training medical students. Currently, Dr. Kim co-chairs the Awards Committee for the Division I (Education in the Professions) of the American Educational Research Association.

**Her colleagues in the School of Medicine:**
> **Doug Brock**, Ph.D. trained in Personality and Social Psychology who has been funded by the Centers for Disease Control to design computer-based and web-based educational applications.
>
> **Thomas Gallagher**, M.D., an internist trained in Medical History & Ethics and a previous Robert Wood Johnson Clinical Scholar who has been funded by the Agency for Healthcare Research and Quality and the Greenwall Foundation to research the communication dimensions of conflicts of interest, research ethics, and disclosure of medical errors and adverse events.
>
> **Carolyn Prouty**, D.V.M, is a veterinarian-turned-researcher examining patient care errors and end of life communication issues.
>
> **Lynne Robins**, Ph.D., a researcher of the effects of physician communication behaviors on patient health outcomes who has designed curricula to promote patient safety, the assessment of clinical competency, cultural competence, and interpersonal communication skills.

**Her colleague in the School of Nursing:**
> **Sarah E. Shannon**, Ph.D., RN, funded by the Agency for Healthcare Research and Quality to study error reduction in rural hospitals and by the National Institute of Nursing Research to test possible improvement in the care of the dying patient in the intensive care unit.

**Her colleague in the School of Pharmacy:**
> **Peggy Odegard**, Pharm.D, CDE, BCPS, the Director of the Geriatrics Program and a Clinical Pharmacy Specialist and Certified Diabetes Educator who researches communication aspects of diabetes and pharmacist interventions.

Thanks to all of you for sharing this amazing example of an on-line case based training module.

## The class session and the student group

Our team has been working together for the past year developing content materials for training and assessing health care providers' knowledge, attitudes, and skills in disclosing medical errors to patients and their families. The graduate seminar we present here is based on the team's work and framed in the context of training graduate students in examining the role of technology in learning. This graduate seminar, titled "Survey of Educational Technology" is offered in our College of Education and is typically attended by masters and doctoral students in Education, Nursing and Medicine.

## Background

Most health science educators believe, and we tend to agree, that case-based teaching is an effective instructional method for improving students' critical thinking skills, decision-making skills and acquisition of content knowledge. When case based teaching is done well, students are challenged to analyze problems presented in cases, make inferences based on limited information, and make decisions on uncertain, ambiguous, and conflicting sets of issues that simulate a real professional context. But in spite of the long history of using cases for training purposes in many academic disciplines including medicine, there is a paucity of scientific evidence for how best to design, use, and evaluate cases for use in curricula. In addition, there is little research on the benefits of this method of teaching with cases in comparison to taking a more didactic approach. With the growing importance of the Web-based case teaching, the need is particularly acute for developing the knowledge base in computer-based case design and for evaluating these curricular offerings. In developing this course we had both of these goals in mind.

## Our Learning Goals and Objectives

The overall goal of this session is for students to explore and examine Web-based case teaching modules that incorporate case design principles identified from the literature and that optimize Web features for enhancing interactivity on the part of the learner. Students are expected to gain an appreciation of how theory guides practice and how practice advances theory using case-based teaching as an example. Students are asked to critically examine the role of technology in instruction with a focus on trainees in the professions of multiple disciplines.

This year, the course focuses on applying case-teaching methods in the development of Web-based case materials. We are using an existing mock-up version of Web-based case modules for students to view and analyze from the theoretical perspective of case-based learning.

An equally important goal for this course is for students to strengthen their critical thinking skills. The analysis of curricula and its effective transformation to an on line, Web based, technology supported offering that facilitates student learning requires high level critical thinking. We want our students to be equipped, at least at the novice level, with the ability to produce their own case based curricular materials at the end of the course. Actually, our goal is even more difficult to accomplish, but not more ambitious than what should be achieved by strong graduate training programs in professional education. We want our students to develop the ability to create materials that foster critical thinking in other health care and educational professionals.

**Learning objectives:**

1. At the end of this session, students will be able to describe recommended case design principles that promote critical thinking skills, particularly methods for making case content engaging and challenging for learners.

2. Using an example of Web-based video cases simulating health care providers' discussions of a medical error, students will be able to discuss Web enabled features that best deliver a sense of realism and immersion from learners' perspectives.

3. Students will develop a mock-up version of Web-based cases that illustrate case development principles and interface design targeting critical thinking abilities in trainees.

**How we teach this Lesson:**

This exercise is carefully designed and deeply layered to assure that students understand the theory behind teaching with online cases. The topics involve providing the background theory, providing an actual experience of an interactive Web case, and guiding the evaluation of the case using the theoretical principles we propose for case design.

**A. Theoretical Framework**

First, students are introduced to the theoretical background of case development. The conceptual framework is developed from a review of 100 reports from multiple disciplines including business, dentistry, education, engineering, law, medicine, and nursing (Kim et al., 2006). Figure 1 summarizes five main dimensions (real, realistic, engaging, challenging, and instructional) and their associated strategies applicable to developing cases.

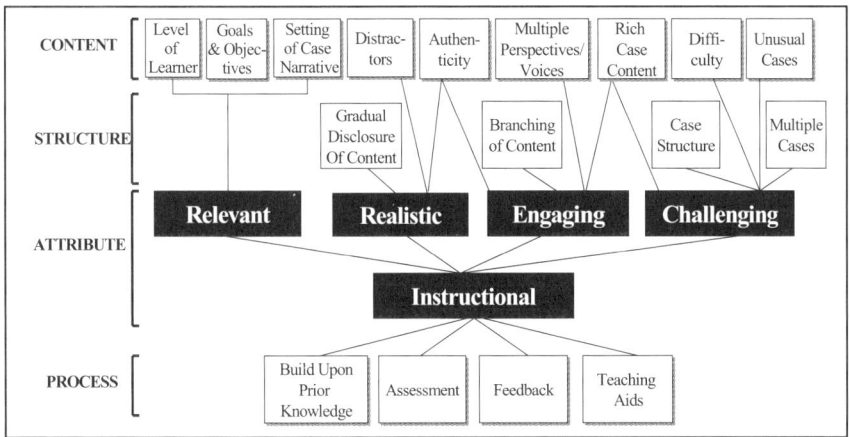

Figure 1: Theoretical Framework of Case Development

Reprinted with permission from Kim et al., 'A conceptual framework for developing teaching cases: a review and synthesis of the literature across disciplines' (2006), *Medical Education,* Vol. 40, pg 869, Blackwell Publishing.

For example, for cases to be relevant to students' needs, the content should
  (a) target an appropriate level of learners;
  (b) match both faculty's and students' goals; and
  (c) specify the setting of the narrative to help students know how to relate to the story.

The level of student engagement is increased when cases
  (a) include rich content to facilitate students' exploration of the situation, characters, and their interactions;
  (b) present multiple voices and perspectives of parties involved in the situation;
  (c) use a branching feature to show different consequences associated with students' decisions.

For cases to have instructional value, the content should
  (a) build upon students' prior knowledge;
  (b) offer multiple cases for students to practice target skills so that their learning can transfer to novel situations;
  (c) incorporate an assessment method to measure students' learning;
  (d) provide specific and corrective feedback; and
  (e) offer teaching aids, such as branching diagrams to support decision-making, case-related questions to stimulate critical thinking, and expert modeling of problem-solving approaches.

## B. Review of a Web Case Example

Following the discussion of the theoretical framework, we have students read and discuss the publication of a recent study (Kim et al., 2007) that applied these case development principles to evaluating Web-based medical cases. For the purposes of the study, Web sites were selected from a pool of Web cases developed for training medical students, residents, and practicing physicians. The study found a minimum use of interactive features in the majority of web sites reviewed. Students are invited to discuss how the lack of interactive features on these sites might compromise trainees' meaningful gains from the posted learning materials.

Next, students will be given a demonstration of a mock-up version of a Web case module that was designed as part of an on-going grant study.

### A sample case scenario is as follows:

"You have admitted a diabetic patient to the hospital for COPD exacerbation. You handwrite an order for the patient to receive "10 U" of insulin. The "U" in your order looks like a 0. The following morning, the patient is given 100 U of insulin, 10 times the patient's normal dose, and is later found unresponsive, with a serum glucose level of 35 mg/DL (1.94 mmol/L). The patient is resuscitated and transferred to the intensive care unit. You expect the patient to make a full recovery" (Gallagher et al., 2006).

The Web case modules deal with a disclosure of medical errors to patients and families by health care providers, and we use this topic in our seminar cases. There are multiple levels of knowledge, attitude, and skills that health care providers, such as physicians, nurses, and pharmacists, need to acquire in order to participate in an effective discussion around medical errors. Here are some of the skills involved:

- recognize that an error has taken place
- define the nature of the error
- assume responsibility for the error
- consider the perspectives of other health care providers on the team
- recognize and respond to less than desirable team interaction dynamics, should they arise
- develop a plan for communicating the cause and implications of the error with patients and families
- handle unanticipated reactions from team members and patients during disclosure

While 'recognition' is often considered a low level skill, it actually entails a high level of reasoning skill in novel or emergent situations. Assessing the situation and determining how to intervene involves the critical thinking skills of analysis, inference, and explanation, and a well made judgment in this situation requires the disposition to honestly evaluate the likelihood of potential consequences of any actions (or inactions). Completing the case well requires the students to anticipate and to prepare to address unforeseen challenges that might arise during the team discussion of the event or during the actual disclosure of an error to a patient. In addition to strong critical thinking, the skilled disclosure of medical errors requires strength in communication. This is regarded as a sophisticated skill in a health care provider. Our educational research project, funded by the Agency for Healthcare Research and Quality, aims to train health care providers in this wide range of skills involved in error disclosure communication.

The Web mock-up cases are media rich and so we are not able to demonstrate all of the case materials here, but the cases use the following interface design elements: (a) segmented video cases which simulate discussions of a medical error among team members and with a patient; (b) embedded questions prompting trainees to provide rationales for their actions; (c) case scenarios of increasing difficulty levels to challenge trainees; and (d) interactive features to engage trainees with case materials. Using the Adobe Flash Player technology, segments of video clips are presented to trainees with various questions associated with each clip. Figure 2 and Figure 3 are sample screenshots from this mock-up case.

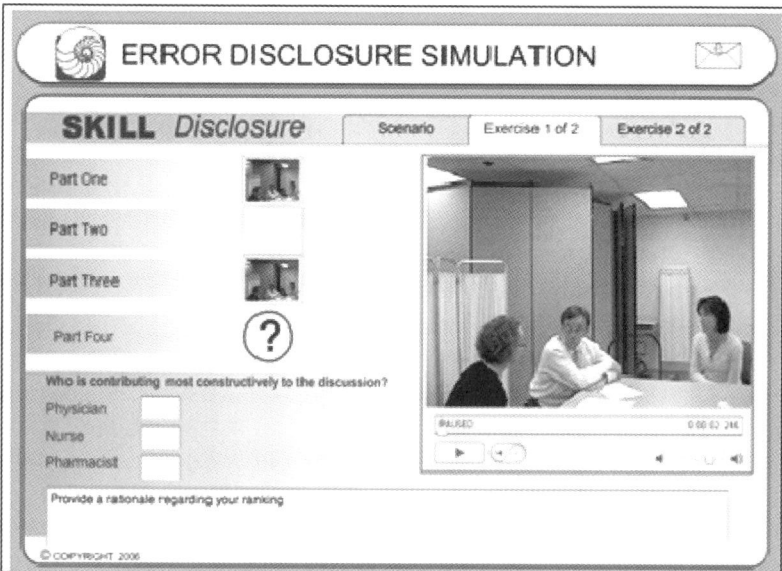

Figure 2: Error Disclosure Simulation Screen Shot A

After selecting an answer to the question, "Who is contributing most constructively to the discussion?" the trainees are prompted to explain the reasoning behind their actions using open-ended text as a way to demonstrate higher-level critical thinking skills. Asking someone to explain 'why' is the most central strategy to increasing the critical thinking component in any class session. In this case students provide evidence of their thinking in the box at the bottom of the frame (Figure 2).

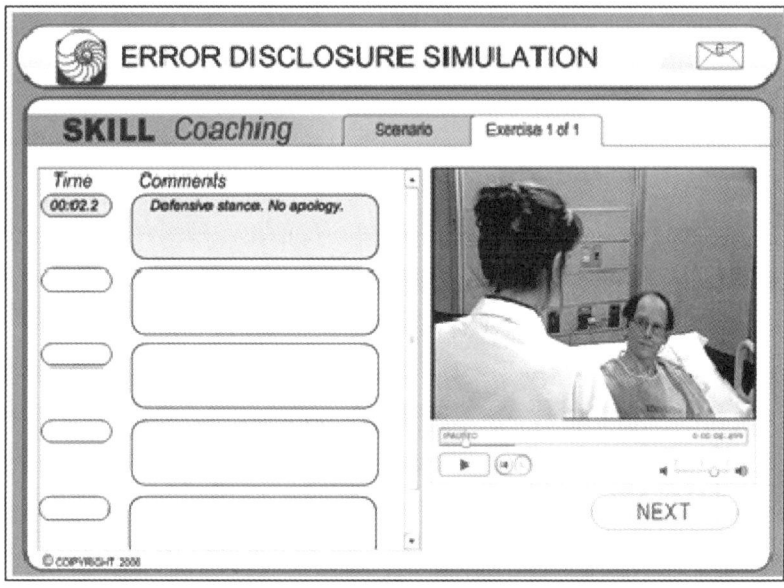

Figure 3: Error Disclosure Simulation Screen Shot B

In Figure 3, the screen shot illustrates a video clip simulating a health care provider making a disclosure to a patient regarding a medical error. Trainees are instructed to put themselves in the role of a coach and provide timely and appropriate feedback to the health care provider portrayed in the video. To do that, they need to be able to interact with the video scenario. This is facilitated by enabling the trainees to pause the clip whenever feedback seems necessary, enter the timestamp linked to the clip, and type their feedback in the space next to the timestamp.

When we examine these typed entries we are able to see how students analyzed and evaluated the words and actions of the provider portrayed in the video and how they themselves might have responded to the scenario in real time. Before the students are asked to evaluate the teaching and learning strengths of this method of Web based case scenarios, it's important that they first experience the case example themselves. When they are asked to evaluate the effectiveness of the Web mock up case, they can use their own learning experience as relevant data.

After viewing the demo, students are invited to discuss the following questions:

1. To what degree are case development principles integrated in this Web mock-up case?

2. Do the interface design features used in this case effectively translate case development principles and help achieve an engaging learning experience?

3. What additional interface design features would you recommend for further development?

4. If you were asked to revise this mock-up version, what would be your main recommendations?

5. In what way do you think the theory needs to be further refined in case development for improving critical thinking skills?

## What I expect from the class participants:

We anticipate that students will complete assigned readings and come to this session well prepared to discuss how theory and practice intersect as illustrated in this example of case teaching principles and designing Web-based interactive cases. Our students are typically fully engaged in the class discussions. Later they develop the ability to demonstrate their own mock-up Web cases and to defend the development of these using the theoretical framework.

## The Student work product:

Students develop and present to the class their version of a mock-up Web case. In the presentation they are expected to articulate the educational values of the interface design features they propose in their mock-up products. We encourage feedback about this class exercise, asking students to reflect back on key learning points they acquired and suggestions for improving the session.

## References:

Gallagher, T.H., Garbutt, J.M., Waterman, A.D., Flum, D.R., Larson, E.B., Waterman, B.M., Dunagan, W.C., Fraser, V.J., & Levinson, W. (2006).Choosing Your Words Carefully:

How Physicians Would Disclose Harmful Medical Errors to Patients. *Archives of Internal Medicine*, 166, 1585-1593.

Kim, S., Phillips, W.R., Pinsky, L., Brock, D.M., Phillips, K., & Keary, J. (2006). A conceptual framework for developing teaching cases: A review and synthesis of literature across disciplines. *Medical Education*, 40, 867-76.

Kim, S., Phillips, W. R.., Huntington, J., Astion, M. L., Keerbs, A., Pinsky, L., Dresden, G., Sharma, U., & Shearer, D.W. (2007). Medical Case Teaching on the Web: Principles, Strategies and Examples. *Teaching and Learning in Medicine* 2007 19(2), 1-9.

**Acknowledgment:**

We would like to acknowledge the following colleagues who collaborated on the conceptual work in case development: Dr. William Phillips, Department of Family Medicine, University of Washington, Dr. Linda Pinsky, Department of Internal Medicine, University of Washington, Ms. Kathryn Phillips, National Business Group on Health, Washington, D.C., and Ms. Jane Keary, Children's Hospital, Seattle, Washington. Also, we thank Mr. Alan Gojdics and Mr. Brian Beardsley in the School of Nursing at University of Washington for their time and effort in creating the mock-up version of the error disclosure Web modules.

# An Analytical and Evaluative Approach to Community-Based Cancer Screening and Prevention projects

## *Noreen C. Facione*

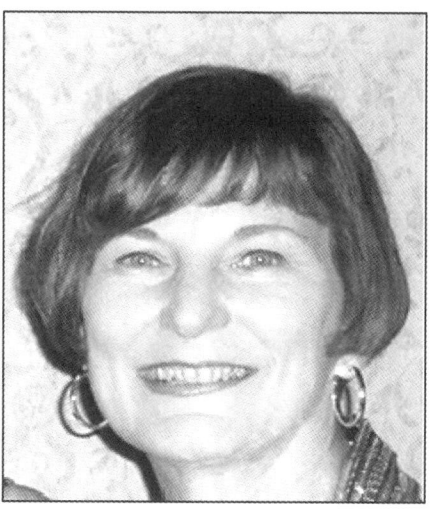

*I will always celebrate the renewed focus on training clinical reasoning skills in our increasingly demanding programs of health science education. Assessing competence in reasoning should be as fundamental as assessing knowledge development. The availability of increasingly powerful medical and surgical treatment is dangerous in the hands of a clinician who has wrongly identified the clinical problem and lacks the ability to analyze and explain a patient's response to treatment. As a result, individuals with very poor reasoning skills should be counseled from our programs early in their training. The others should be continually practiced in case analysis and be asked to voice the reasoned explanation of their planned clinical interventions according to their advancing competence.*

*This lesson prepared clinicians and graduate level students to design a targeted community based cancer screening project and then to evaluate it in terms of its productivity for advancing cancer early detection. Set in the context of practice, it focuses on evidenced based program planning and evaluation. This exercise of critical thinking skills and habits of mind generalizes well to other aspects of the clinical role and to other community based projects.*

## Introduction

In the mid 1990's health science education programs adjusted their curricula to include an emphasis on health promotion and illness prevention and medical centers began to focus on delivering prevention and early detection programs to the community outside the Medical Center walls. As a member of the oncology nursing faculty at UC San Francisco, I had the opportunity to prepare a new course for graduate level students on cancer epidemiology, screening and prevention. I seized this opportunity to bring my research findings to the classroom, realizing that in preparing health science clinicians for clinical practice I was educating those who would one day be responsible for recommending participation in cancer screening or even designing and implementing community outreach programs. My goal was for students to learn how to design community based early detection projects with clear and obtainable objectives, well-estimated benefit to the community, fiscal responsibility, and an evaluation plan for assessing actual benefit to the community. The goal fit well with another always present goal in my teaching: helping students to develop stronger clinical reasoning skills.

**Session overview**

The lesson is designed in three sections, each targeting difference critical thinking skills or dispositional foci. During the first hour of the session, participants analyze cancer incidence and mortality statistics by population group and review cancer screening guidelines and prevention recommendations (Section 1). In the second, they design a targeted community-based project supported by inferences and explanations developed out of their analyses of most at risk populations in their community (Section 2). The last hour is a fair-minded evaluation of a completed cancer screening or prevention project (Section 3), either one that they carried out themselves or one that has been published in the literature. Whether this offering is conducted as a staff development workshop or as a component of a graduate seminar, it is best held either as a three hour emersion experience or as three, sequential, one hour sessions.

Section 1 could be shortened or omitted, in the interest of time, if the participants have a working knowledge of cancer incidence and prevalence, recommended cancer screening guidelines and prevention recommendations, and known cultural barriers to cancer prevention and detection. However, Section 1 offers the opportunity to set the stage for a systematic analysis of cancer prevalence, at-risk populations, and the necessity for an evidence-based and culturally competent matched response in the planned project.

**Session participants**

This session outlines a segment of a multidisciplinary elective course designed for clinical programs in the health sciences, public health, health care economics, and health care ethics. It has also been offered as a three hour continuing education workshop for practicing clinicians to refresh their awareness of the current cancer burden and current community based efforts at early detection. The model for this session would generalize to training sessions for those who have the responsibility for developing and evaluating community outreach programs.

## Learning objectives

There are multiple critical thinking focused learning objectives for the three hour session. The final summative objective calls for an evidence based clinical judgment about the value of the evaluated cancer screening or prevention project:

> **Section 1:**
> a) Accurately analyze and interpret cancer incidence and mortality data to identify an appropriate target population (analysis) and to identify either prevention or early detection objectives for their community-based project (inference and explanation).
>
> **Section 2:**
> b) Design a community based cancer screening project (inference and explanation) to address these objectives.
>
> **Section 3:**
> c) Evaluate an actual cancer screening or prevention project against some standard or criterion for cancer control (analysis and evaluation; systematicity and cognitive maturity).
>
> d) Make a fair-minded, evidence-based judgment about the value of a completed cancer screening or prevention project (interpretation, analysis and evaluation; truth-seeking, open-mindedness).

## Material used for the session

Section 1 of this lesson calls for the interpretation and analysis of a large array of documents and data reports. These will have to be made available to participants. Projection of Internet-based graphics to big screen or desktop/laptop display is an environmentally conscious approach to this requirement. The list includes:

- United States data from the Center for Disease Control on cancer incidence and mortality. These data are annually summarized for clinicians on the Centers for Disease Control website www.cdc.gov and presented as *Cancer Facts and Figures* on the American Cancer Society (ACS) website www.cancer.org. These statistics are provided by the Center for Disease Control U.S. Cancer Statistics Working Group (2007) and updated annually.

- Cancer screening guidelines and cancer prevention recommendations. My preferred source is the National Cancer Institute (NIH) website which posts current guidelines for each cancer site: http://www.cancer.gov/cancerinfo/screening. They also provide a research based discussion of the likely effectiveness of cancer prevention and early detection efforts. See for example their comments on two lung cancer screening approaches, noting both strengths and weaknesses. Other guidelines are available on the web, for example the Canadian Task Force on Preventive Health Care Recommendations and the American Academy of Family Physicians Task Force Report.

Sections 2 and 3 call for the design and evaluation of a community based cancer screening project. I make these available by electronic projection and suggest that participants conduct additional electronic literature searches as well.

- Published reports of community based cancer early detection programs. These are retrievable with a literature search of digital library resources.

## Section One: analyze cancer incidence and mortality statistics by population group

Perhaps the best effect of the new emphasis on evidence based practice is the call for a clear explanation and evaluation of clinical action based on observable data. Implicit is the need to analyze the clinical situation, develop a clear and consensus description of the problem, and identify which data would provide a relevant explanation or evaluation in each practice circumstance. Incidence and mortality data are always four or five years old, due to the time needed for compilation, but they can be examined for differences by age, sex, geographical area, and racial and ethnic background. When these data are well interpreted and analyzed, they provide evidence of at risk and potentially underserved populations, as well as a basis for setting community outreach program priorities in relationship to United States cancer incidence and mortality. I begin by examining some of the available graphic presentations aloud to model a systematic review, analyzing trends in relationship to past screening practices and connecting the graphic with an explanation of what is known about cancer predisposition, age at presentation and available screening modalities. I have found that I can reliably assume that many students and fellow clinicians will not have the habit of mind of being thorough in their analyses. Figures 1 and 2 provide examples of the type of graphics that could be used in the Section 1 analysis discussion to determine which cancer sites might be addressed in a community based screening project and which populations should be targeted. Talking aloud while conducting a thoughtful and fair-minded analysis of this type of data nurtures the critical thinking dispositions of truth-seeking, inquisitiveness and systematicity and the skills of analysis and inference. These cognitive behaviors are also easily generalizable to other clinical reasoning situations.

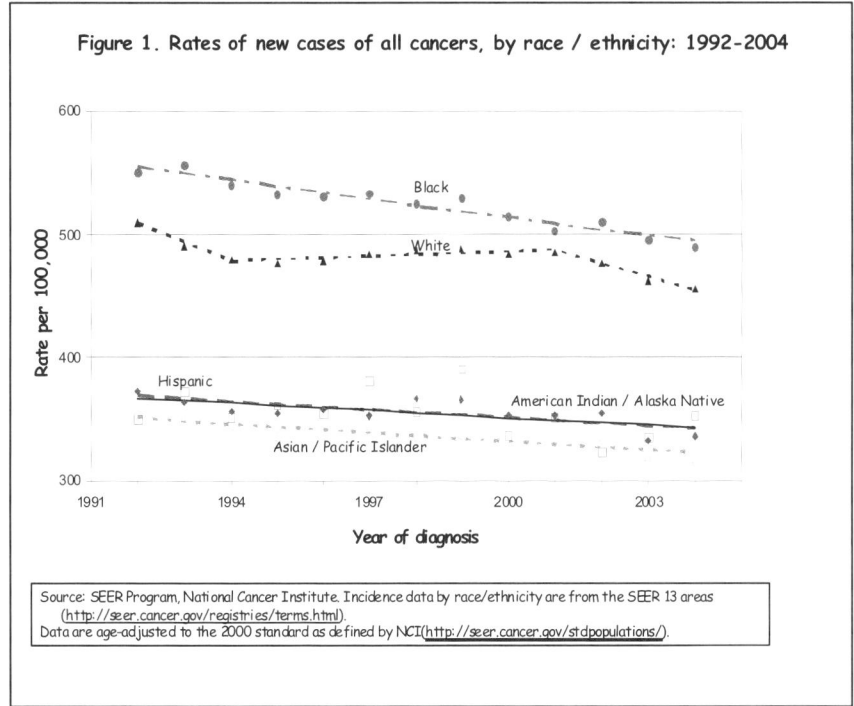

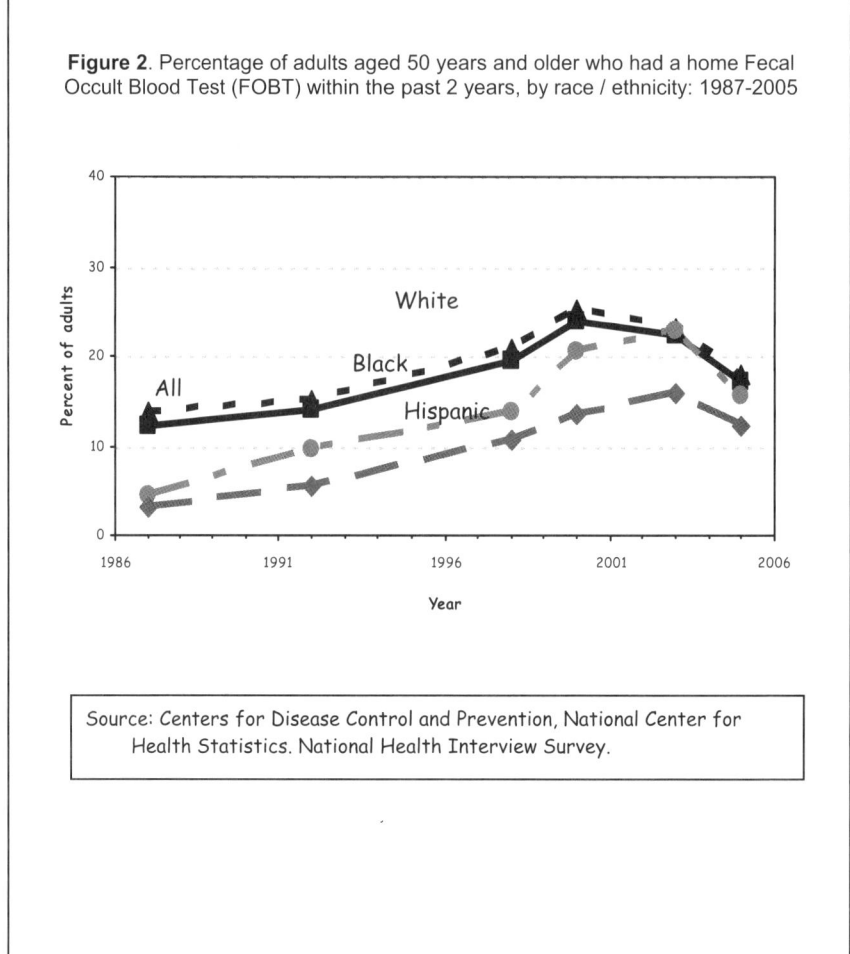

**Figure 2**. Percentage of adults aged 50 years and older who had a home Fecal Occult Blood Test (FOBT) within the past 2 years, by race / ethnicity: 1987-2005

Source: Centers for Disease Control and Prevention, National Center for Health Statistics. National Health Interview Survey.

## Section Two: Design of a Cancer Screening Project

The particular cancer focus of the cancer screening or prevention project is not in itself important, but I usually encourage session participants to begin by considering the design of a screening for prostate, breast, colorectal cancer or melanoma because of their prevalence. Some will also want to attempt to impact lung cancer deaths and will need to evaluate approaches to screening versus prevention (smoking cessation) projects. An appropriate choice of smoking cessation should result from the analyses in Section1 which should have uncovered information like that included in Figure 3.

*An Analytical and Evaluative Approach to Community-Based Projects*

---

**Figure 3: Lung Cancer Screening Modalities**

1) Screening for Lung Cancer with Chest X-Ray and/or Sputum Cytology
- Benefits Screening does not reduce mortality from lung cancer (fair evidence).
- Harms Screening would lead to false-positive tests and unnecessary invasive diagnostic procedures and treatments (solid evidence).
- <u>Description of the Evidence</u>: Randomized controlled trials with fair internal validity due to lack of unscreened groups and contamination. No evidence of effect. External validity of the findings is fair, due to lack of women and minority groups. False-positive results range from 4% to 15%; there is a possibility of over-diagnosis and overtreatment (magnitude uncertain).

2) Screening for Lung Cancer with Low-Dose Helical Computed Tomography (LDCT)
- Benefits The evidence is inadequate to determine whether screening reduces mortality from lung cancer.
- Harms Screening would lead to false-positive tests and unnecessary invasive diagnostic procedures and treatments (solid evidence).
- Description of the Evidence: Cohort or case-control studies with poor internal validity for answering the question of mortality reduction. The magnitude of the effect cannot determine from the available studies. False-positive results range from 20% to 50%; over-diagnosis and overtreatment are possible (magnitude uncertain).

---

Small group work (4 to 5 clinicians or students) optimizes both the information available to plan the project and the communication of the thinking process behind the project design. The consideration of culturally relevant outreach, the particular experience of each screening test, potential false positive and false negative screening test rates, the necessity of following up on positive screening tests, and related strategic issues and financial costs is expected to be a part of this project design. Group members are guided to explain their analyses and inferences by a short session guideline I provide (Figure 5). The recommendation of a one hour timeline for Section 2 implies that the session participants have well established group discussion skills. I don't favor assigning a group leader in this type of exercise as they tend to stifle the thinking process. I make rounds on the groups, limiting my comments to asking questions that ask the group to clarify the assumptions being made and the logical connections that should be implicit in the project. At times I need to challenge a groups' assumptions with published findings (capitalizing on teaching from my area of expertise) or point out potential bias or stereotyping of population groups.

---

**Figure 4. Prevention or early detection project**

- cancer site (data supported)
- at risk population (data supported)
- optimal screening modalities
- benefits (study supported)
- potential harms (study supported)
- prevention recommendations (National guidelines)
- prevention or detection goals for this project
- cultural/demographic considerations
- potential strategic barriers (drawn from the literature)
- project personnel
- action plan and timeline
- screening plan and follow-up
- prevention plan and follow-up
- project evaluation plan (with brief rationale)
- project budget (with brief rationale)

---

***Written work product for Section 2:*** In the context of a workshop for clinicians where we will quickly move on to Section 3, I ask each group to prepare a two page summary that covers the points in Figure 4. If this part of the exercise will be used to design an actual cancer prevention or screening project, the length of the report might best take the format of an intramural small grant application. In all cases the length of the discussion of the proposed project should be short and require the writer to be concise and clear, and to supply the evidence base for all key considerations and judgments. This type of requirement forces the write to reanalyze the thinking behind each portion of the project planning in order to present it well in the short summary or finding proposal.

### Section Three: evaluation of a completed cancer screening project

Even good thinkers sometimes hold on to poorly made (or even life-threatening) decisions, refusing to reconsider. Past practices are continued in the absence of evaluation. So it's never too soon to subject a practice, a judgment or a favorite project to a fair-minded critical analysis. So I remind participants that it is always appropriate to ask whether goals have been met, or for the reasons behind a continuing effort. In this case we are asking "Should we fund other cancer screening or prevention projects like this one?" Ideally the participants should be evaluating a project that they have conducted, as a way of assessing the benefits and harms of the project and the evidence for continuing it into the future. However, often the time available does not support this ideal and instead Section 3 involves the evaluation of a published report of a community-based cancer screening or prevention program conducted elsewhere.

Possessing ability in critical thinking (skills) is no guarantee of possessing the mental discipline use these skills (disposition) to address critical clinical situations using a critical thinking approach. Knowing this I try never to pass up an opportunity to model both. In this case I talk aloud through the evaluation of a cancer screening or prevention project, covering all of the areas I will expect the participants to cover in their own project evaluation. These are outlines in Figure 5.

You may want to locate and provide written reports for use in this portion of the lesson, particularly when time is of the essence. This literature is uneven in quality, many reports being full of unsupported claims of success in reaching cancer control goals. When time permits, more learning occurs when participants are asked to locate the report individually. The most common error in locating a project to evaluate occurs when participants locate a report of an on-going national project that has yet to be completed or evaluated. In this case they have no way to evaluate the claims of the authors as to the project's benefit. I've found that I frequently need to assist weaker thinkers to identify an appropriate published report that fits the criteria of the exercise and provides them adequate information to respond to the assignment. I keep a list of recent papers reporting on neighborhood screening programs, some of which are included in the references. These are easier to approach and analyze than reports of National screening programs, yet they offer an adequate challenge, and they are more informative to future local efforts at cancer control.

***Written or presented work product for Section 3:*** Once again, while the expected breadth of this written evaluation is considerable, the length of the written response should necessarily be short. This is because executives in the workplace rarely read long reports. It's best to train efforts to present the results of a strong critical thinking process in a concise report. Bullet lists might even be included to summarize key points and supportive evidence where appropriate, much as has been done in this chapter. Figure 5 provides a structure for the evaluation.

> **Figure 5. Evaluation Guidelines for Cancer Screening or Prevention Project**
> - Evaluate each of the following:
> - overall project goals in relationship to established National cancer control goals (e.g. Goals 2010)
> - the selection of cancer site and chosen target population
> - the selection of and actual provision of cancer prevention or screening control activities
> - the expected benefits and harms
> - the use and adequacy of project personnel
> - the justification of cost
> - the cultural competence of project activities
> - the efforts to overcome known strategic barriers
> - the actual (benefits and harms) contribution made by this project to cancer control for this community
> - Provide a brief comment as to the basis for each area of evaluation.

## Comments on the cultural relevance

Perhaps you have been thinking, "This type of evaluation exercise would not be culturally appropriate in my country because this type of evaluation is carried out by only a few." It is true that the expectation of a voiced evaluation of existing programs will differ by country and even by cultural group within a country. In the United States we both value a well thought out critique of common practice or a particular project, and we have the freedom to express it in most circumstances. Even with this freedom, the evaluation is rarely appreciated or headed unless it is presented in a logically well-framed and evidenced-based manner. But even in situations where one may not have either the freedom or the privilege of expressing the results of an informed evaluation, the ability to carry out an internal critical thinking process resulting in a sound evaluation that can inform one's practice is usually prized. *Those who have practiced skills in fair-minded evaluation are the source of future leadership.*

Thus, regardless of the cultural practices regarding the expected source of a voiced evaluation, I would suggest that all staff development programs and health science educational programs offer lessons like this one that practice the critical thinking skills and dispositions necessary to evaluate practice guidelines, on-going programs and the results of new initiatives.

## Assessment data

An examination of performance on this assignment, using some qualitative criteria or a rubric, like the Holistic Critical Thinking Scoring Rubric (HCTSR),* will provide a measure of the groups' ability to think critically about an authentic workplace issue. The written reports produced in Sections 2 and 3 also provide excellent portfolio data to assess the groups' overall capability to think critically.

## References

American Academy of Family Physicians. Summary of policy recommendations for periodic health examination. Retrieved September 19, 2000, from the World Wide Web: http://www.aafp.org/exam.xml.

Canadian Task Force on Preventive Health Care. CTFPHC Systematic reviews and recommendations. Retrieved March 13, 2000, from the World Wide Web: http://www.ctfphc.org.

Crane, L. A., Leakey, T. A., Rimer, B. K., Wolfe, P., Woodworth, M. A., & Warnecke, R. B. (1998). Effectiveness of a telephone outcall intervention to promote screening mammography among low-income women. *Preventive Medicine*, 27, S39-S49.

Fitzgibbon, M. L., Stolley, M. R., Avellone, M. E., Chavez, N, & Sugerman, S. (1996). Involving parents in cancer risk reduction: A program for Hispanic American families. *Health Psychology*, 15(6), 413-422.

Lechner, L., deVries, H., & Offermans, N. (1997). Participation in a breast cancer screening program: Influence of a past behavior and determinants on future screening participation. Preventive Medicine, 26, 473-483.

Mettlin C., Murphy, G. P., Babalan, R. J., Chesley, A., Kane, R. A., Littrup, P. J., Mostoff, F. K., Ray, P. S., Shanberg, A. M., & Toi, A. (1996). The results of a five year early prostate cancer detection intervention. *Cancer*, 77(1), 150-159.

Resnicow, K., Royce, J., Vaughn, R., Orlandi, M. A., and Smith, M. (1997). Analysis of a multicomponent smoking cessation project: What worked and why? Preventive Medicine, 26, 373-381.

SEER Cancer Statistics Review, 1975-2003 (NCI) http://seer.cancer.gov/csr/1975_2003

Sung, J. F., Blumenthal, D. S., Coates, R. J., Williams, J. E., Alema-Mensah, E., and Liff, J. M. (1997). Effect of a cancer screening intervention conducted by lay health workers among inner city women. *American Journal of Preventive Health*, 13(1), 51-57.

Tilley, B.C., Vernon, S.W., Glanz, K., Myers, R., Sanders, K., Lu M., Hirst, K., Kristal, A. R., Smereka, C., & Sowers, M.F. (1997). Worksite cancer screening and nutrition intervention for high risk auto workers: Design and baseline findings of the next step trial. *Preventive Medicine*, 26, 227-235.

Urban, N., Taplin, S. H., Taylor, V. M., Peacock, S., Anderson, G., Conrad, D., Etzioni, R., White, E., Montano, D. E., Mahlock, J., & Majer, K. (1995). Community organization to promote breast cancer screening among women ages 50-75. *Preventive Medicine*, 24, 477- 484.

U.S. Cancer Statistics Working Group. *United States Cancer Statistics:* 1999–2004 *Incidence and Mortality Web-based Report.* Atlanta: U.S. Department of Health and Human Services, Centers for Disease Control and Prevention *and* National Cancer Institute; 2007. Available at: www.cdc.gov/uscs.

Weinrich, S.P., Boyd, M.D., Bradford, D., Mossa, M.S. & Weinrich, M. (1998). Recruitment of African Americans into prostate cancer screening. *Cancer Practice*, 6(1),23-30.

---

* In the last chapter in this volume Peter Facione – with whom I co-authored the HCTSR in 1994, shares one of his favorite rubric exercises. There he provides a copy of the HCTSR and instructions for its use.

# Advocating Through the Media: Cultivating CT Dispositions in a Distance-Learning Course

## *Mary M. Hoke & Leslie K. Robbins*

*Drs. Mary Hoke [right] and Leslie Robbins [below] are colleagues in the School of Nursing at New Mexico State University. Both are advanced practice nurses who advocate for interactive learning strategies. They have facilitated the education of nursing students with a variety of cultural and ethnic backgrounds in all levels of nursing education. This chapter describes a lesson that engages students' critical thinking skills, but here the authors stress that their focus is most on cultivating critical thinking habits of mind.*

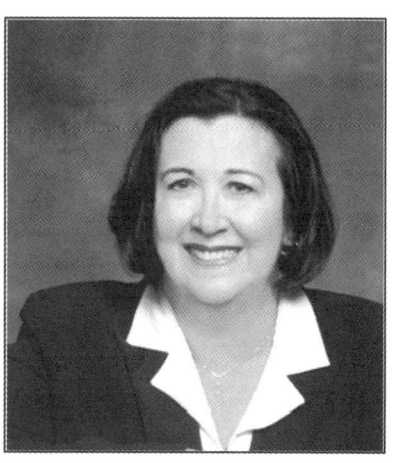

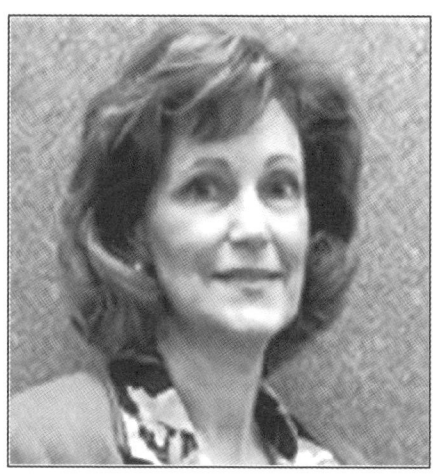

*We agree with these authors that it is highly important to remember to cultivate a critical thinking disposition. Recent models of human reasoning describe two interactive cognitive systems (one pre-reflective and holistic and the other analytical and evaluative) that balance and check each other when humans think well (see more on this in our introductory chapter). Without a critical thinking disposition, one might imagine underutilization of the analytical and evaluative system and too much unchecked reliance on pre-reflective holistic judgments. So we hope you will enjoy this discussion of building the critical thinking dispositions of analyticity, critical thinking self-confidence, and cognitive maturity.*

*The description of how this class is conducted is nothing short of marvelous! This lesson is taught simultaneously in three settings using distance learning capability. Students are managed in small group discussions, a highly authentic, largely unrehearsed and relevant communication exercise and a self-evaluation debrief. This is a great example of the type of daring pedagogy that makes for excellence in teaching even under distance learning constraints. This work was funded in part by the Health Resources and Services Administration (HRSA), United States Department of Health and Human Services.*

## An introduction to the class session

We teach this lesson in a course entitled "Issues and Trends" that is part of our Bachelor of Science in Nursing Completion Program. Our goal for this class session is to enlarge nursing students' advocacy skills through effective utilization of various media outlets. Engaging in this class exercise builds our students' critical thinking disposition. In describing critical thinking disposition, we use the terminology introduced by the American Philosophical Association Delphi Study by Dr. Peter Facione (APA, 1990). The critical thinking dispositions identified in this study were later replicated by the researchers at Pennsylvania State University (Jones and Ratcliff, 1994) and used to create a measurement tool (Facione & Facione, 1996). In this lesson we are working to develop all of the critical thinking dispositions when the opportunity arises, but we have focused our learning objectives particularly on analyticity, critical thinking (CT) self-confidence, and cognitive maturity.

## The students

The students in this course are already licensed to practice as registered nurses and have an Associate Degree or Diploma from previous study in nursing at another school or college. They have returned to school to obtain a higher degree that typically includes courses building advanced content knowledge, professionalism, leadership, ethics, research utilization, and communication skills.

## Learning objectives and the associated critical thinking dispositions that are the focus for each

Students who participate in this class session will be able to:
1. Accurately articulate news worthy messages for current nursing issues (cognitive maturity, CT self-confidence).

2. Demonstrate effective communication skills when interacting with the media (analyticity, CT self-confidence).

3. Assess advocacy effectiveness when using radio and television media outlets (cognitive maturity, CT self-confidence.

In achieving these learning objectives the students also practice their critical thinking skills, most notably analysis, inference and evaluation, but we find it helpful to sometimes think only of the dispositions so we do not miss an opportunity to compliment students who demonstrate them.

**Our work before class for this assignment**

New Mexico State University's School of Nursing has distance education capability, and offers courses on our main campus as well as two other satellite sites. We teach this class through both an on-line course software program (providing the capability of posting syllabi, assigned readings, text and/or picture files, slide presentations and the ability for students to communicate through internet postings) and an interactive television capability (ITV) that has larger band width that allows for internet-based interactive audio and video connections from the main campus to two other sites.

Preparation for this class includes assembling props for triads of students; developing and filming a mock interview; and making arrangements to have a media specific video streamed to students through the on-line course software program we use for the class. A symbolic television camera, microphone, and interviewer notepad are gathered for each group of three students. By 'symbolic' we mean that the camera and microphone will not be connected to a live broadcast and the interviewer will not be a member of the actual media. These props, along with any handouts we provide for students during the class session, are prepared and sent to the two distance learning sites before the actual class session.

We prepare the filmed mock interview to last about 10 minutes and to contain a multitude of obviously positive and negative media communications made by the interviewee. The players in the filmed interview include a nurse educator (interviewee) who receives a telephone call requesting an interview later in the day, a reporter from a local television station (interviewer) and a camera technician. We were able to do this with the faculty and staff serving as the actors. Our college's media specialist has been a valuable resource assisting us with the actual filming of this mock media interview.

**How We Teach this Lesson**

Prior to class, students are required to view instructional content related to media relations. We use the American Nurses Association's video "ANA Media

Relations and You." (ANA Media Relations). We ask students to analyze the information in the video to identify guidelines that will assist them in working with media outlets, and to bring their analyses to class. This sets the stage for taking an organized approach to activities within the class session, a demonstration of the critical thinking disposition of systematicity. Specifically, this provides students with an initial framework to assess the quality of the class exercises to follow. The lesson itself is divided into three segments, each with an exercise that develops critical thinking dispositions.

## Segment 1: Analysis of a video interview

During the first segment, the mock interview video is shown to the students. We ask them to watch it individually and to analyze and evaluate the media performance of the nurse educator interviewee, listing positive and negative points within the video. If the class was being conducted at a single site, a live role play mock interview could be provided by faculty instead of the videotape. Following the mock interview, we discuss the students' observations as a group. The instructors' job is to analyze insightful student comments and help students see that these can be summarized by the categories of interview preparation and interview performance (see a brief description of these below).

| Preparation | Performance |
|---|---|
| The Situation | Message |
| • Type of interview/media | • Verbal |
| • Purpose of the interview- subject | • Visual |
| • Length of interview | • Written |
| • What reporter hopes to gain | |
| Your Message | Sender |
| • Major theme-Number of concepts | • Stay in control |
| • Support data (key stats) | • Stay on message |
| • Human interest aspect (personal examples & stories) | • Maintain credibility |
| • Anticipate and prepare for possible questions& formulate responses | • Be mindful of transitions |
| | • Nothing is off the record |
| Yourself | Receiver |
| • Appearance counts | • Significance |
| • Practice | • Sound bites |
| • Quiet time (compose yourself) | • Take away message |
| • Like an job interview (be early & be ready) | |

## Segment 2: The Media Interview

During the second segment of the lesson, each of the students participate in an interview experience, and evaluate that interview experience. To accomplish this, we first divide the students into groups identified as Group A, Group B, or Group C. Then, we ask the A's, B's and C's to divide themselves into groups of no more than 4 students in each group (i.e.: Group A1, Group A2, etc). These letter designations will be used later to assign roles for the interview to follow.

We tell the students the following: "You are nurses at a local hospital and you have just been contacted by the media with the request that you please provide a television interview for your local television station. A reporter will be conducting the interview at the hospital, and they want to do the interview within the next 2 hours. The topic of the interview is the current nursing issue on the paper you are now being given." Then, we give each group a current nursing issue, and we ask each group to develop three talking points with supporting documentation and local examples. Each group is given a different issue from which they are to develop the talking points. Figure 1 provides a list of possible issues we might have used in this lesson this year. The list can change at any time permitting us to maintain clinically relevant content in the lesson.

- Impact of technology on nursing care
- Mental health services in acute care settings
- Physician-nurse games
- Best practices- evidenced based practice
- Short length of stays for new babies/moms
- Cultural practices in death and dying
- Role of clinical nurse leader
- Nursing shortage
- Deaths and disabilities caused by hospitalization/health care
- Emergency preparedness/terrorism
- Emerging communicable disease (West Nile, Hanta, MRSA)
- Domestic violence
- Union representation in nursing
- Least restrictive environment for elders
- Least restrictive environment for mentally ill
- Patient Privacy- HIPAA
- Birth control services for adolescents
- Fetal tissue use (stem cell research)
- Cloning
- Limited malpractice awards

**Figure 1: Sample Issues to Mock Interviews**

Preparing for the interview encourages students to identify and plan for potential problems (analyticity). During the development of talking points and the actual interview that follows we can observe students demonstrating the disposition of CT self-confidence, particularly when they talk aloud about how they will make a particular argument and back it up with sound reasons. We also can see when they lack confidence in this ability. Later when they accomplish the task of making the points in the interview we can reinforce growth in their ability to think while being interviewed. Seeing a student anticipate the consequences of making a particular talking point and role playing possible responses, particularly to controversial issues, is one way we observe students demonstrating the critical thinking disposition of analyticity.

After the students work in their groups to complete the talking points (this takes about 10-15 minutes), we ask the students to restructure their groups into triads, with each triad consisting of one student from Group A, one from Group B, and one from Group C. This new grouping is the one where the interview exercise will be carried out. We have mixed the groups to add a measure of unfamiliarity between the soon to be interviewer and interviewee in the newly constituted groups. We assign the role of interviewee to the student in the group who was a Group A person, the job of interviewer to the previous Group B person and the job of camera technician (observer) to the student who was earlier in Group C. The camera technician is a key role for capturing insights about the interview exercise. This student is asked to watch the interaction, analyzing the media communication and critically evaluating it. They can do this better without the requirement of participating in the interview. Assigning this type of role to a critical observer is typically central to a critical thinking exercise that includes a meta level debriefing at the end. They are also always instructed to be honest and to provide an evidence base for their critique.

Next, each new triad completes a 7-10 minute interview. The student who is the designated interviewee uses their talking points as they are being interviewed. After completion of the interview, the students return to their original small group (A's, B's and C's). Here they share their individual experiences during the interview exercise and assess the quality of the interview, bringing the perspective of their assigned role. They identify positive and negative aspects of the interviews they experienced, much as they did for the video mock interview earlier in the lesson. Finally we ask then to examine each identified negative aspect for possible corrective actions. As with many of our small group exercises, each group selects a spokesperson to report back to the class once the work is completed.

We look for fair-mindedness, open-mindedness and cognitive maturity to be demonstrated when the students evaluate the interview based on their prescribed role and in light of other students' comments. While they are doing this portion of the exercise we are watching and listening. Any student can talk with us through the ITV if they need to clarify the task or resolve an issue. This discussion period usually lasts for about 15-20 minutes.

This second segment of this lesson can be changed to have students rotate roles with different issues, up to three times. The limitation to the number of rotated roles is based on the length of the class session and the number of students in the class. As our class includes interactive television and multiple sites, we make a conscious decision on when and how to include the students at the various sites.

## Segment 3: Building confidence in media skills

During the third and final segment of this lesson, we convene again as a large group across the three settings so that the spokespersons can summarize for the entire class the key findings in their small group and offer any identified corrective actions. It's a necessity that this debriefing session be generally positive and supportive if we are to succeed in our effort to build critical thinking self confidence in these students. So comments identifying weak or negative interview experience points are followed by the successful identification of ways to improve on the next opportunity.

We like to start with group reports from spokespersons who were the interviewer, then move to spokespersons who were interviewees, and finish with spokespersons who were the camera technician/observer spokespersons. As the summarizations are presented, we record key points and later conduct a summary discussion of opportunities to gain local media advocacy experiences, and resources for further support. There are many opportunities in this section of the class to point out and complement students who demonstrate critical thinking skills and the specific dispositions we are hoping to reinforce. One of our jobs is to listen for these and focus our comments on valuing the demonstration of the dispositions.

**Student Work Product**

Most of the work for this lesson occurs in the class but we also ask students to repeat the experience at home by individually selecting a current nursing issue (not one used in today's class), and developing three talking points related to the issue. The components of the talking points are to include a general statement, supporting data, and at least one personal/local example. Students submit this work by posting it in the on-line component of the course within seven days. In addition to well chosen issues and well organized talking points, we look for evidence of critical thinking disposition in these postings.

**Student Feedback**

Many students report that they had not previously seen working with the media as a skill they would/could use in their local areas, but that now they can imagine participating in a media interview (being confident in their thinking process - CT self-confidence). The importance of knowing the key message they wanted to convey was consistently noted (anticipating what happens next - analyticity). Further, the use of the format provided a systematic guide to both prepare for the interview and assist them in identifying the key message when they had lots of information/data (valuing an organized approach - systematicity). Typically students saw the use of the videotaped mock interview combined with practice in class, as providing them with a safe environment to practice media use skills while still having a good time.

**References**

ANA Media Relations & You Toot Kit. Available from American Nurses Association, 600 Maryland Avenue, SW, Suite 100-West, Washington, DC 20024, (202)-651-7028. E-mail: RN=RealNews@ana.org, www.nursingworld.org/rnrealnews

American Philosophical Association (APA). (1990).Critical Thinking: A Statement of Expert Consensus for Purposes of Educational Assessment and Instruction, ("The Delphi Report"). ERIC Doc. No. ED 315-423, pp. 80. The Executive Summary, including tables and recommendations, is available as a free download at www.insightassessment.com.

Facione, N. C. & Facione, P. A. (1996) Externalizing the critical thinking in knowledge development and clinical judgment. *Nursing Outlook*, 44, 129-136.

Hoke, M. M., & Robbins, L.K. (2005). Active Learning's Impact on Nursing Students' Success. *Journal of Holistic Nursing,* 23, 348-355.

Jones, B., & Ratcliff, G. (1994). "Critical Thinking Goals Inventory." United States Department of Education, Office of Educational Research and Improvement, Grant R11760037, CFDA No: 84.117G.

Robbins, L.K., & Hoke, M. M. *(in press)*. OSCEs Promote Development of Clinical and Cultural Competencies for Advanced Practice Psychiatric Mental Health Nursing Students. *Psychiatric Care Perspectives.*

**Acknowledgement**

The process described is supported in part by funds from the Division of Nursing (DN), Bureau of Health Professions (BHPr), Health Resources and Services Administration (HRSA), Department of Health and Human Services (DHHS) under grant number D11HP00440 Southern New Mexico RN to BSN Initiative for $2,456,343 The content and conclusions are those of the authors and should not be construed as the official position or policy of, nor should any endorsements be inferred by the Division of Nursing, BHPr, DHHS or the U.S. Government.

# Unfolding Case Studies: Dynamic Mental Models in a Public Health Context

## *Jo Azzarello*

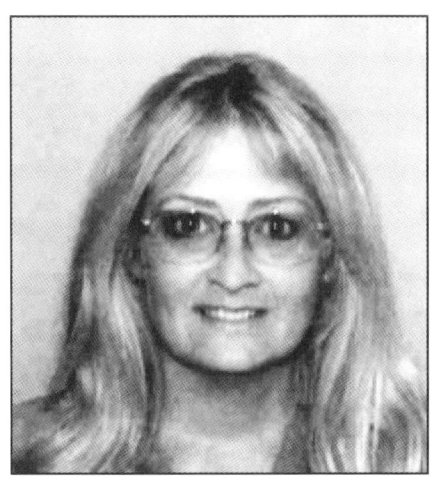

*Dr. Jo Azzarello offers us an opportunity to examine the use of case studies in this example chapter. She is an Associate Professor in the College of Nursing at the University of Oklahoma Health Sciences Center. Her specialty expertise is Diabetes Education and the use of Mental Models and computerized Cognitive Tutors. Dr. Azzarello is an active member of the American Diabetes Association, the Council for the Advancement of Diabetes Research and Education, the Southern Nursing Research Society, Sigma Theta Tau International, and the National League for Nursing.*

*'Mental model' is a term used to describe a person's interpretation of a presenting problem situation. The model might be simple (such as 'the car is speeding') or it might be very complex and involve a great deal of scientific or theoretical information. But the important thing about a mental model is that humans rely on them to determine what they believe and how they will act (Senge, 1990). Dr. Azzarello focuses this lesson on training the ability to adapt one's mental model as one becomes more knowledgeable about the problem situation. Without this ability, one is likely to be working on a suboptimal or inaccurate framing of the problem and arriving at a suboptimal or even incorrect resolution. Adapting one's mental model in the like of new evidence is the result of analysis, inference and explanation and also captures the habit of mind we have identified as the critical thinking disposition of 'cognitive maturity.' This ability is vital to competent clinical reasoning. These are components of problem framing (getting the problem right), a first necessary if subsequent intervention are to be relevant. To supplement the material in this chapter, we also recommend Dr. Azzarello's 2006 paper in Nurse Educator (cited below).*

## Background:

One hallmark of growing expertise is an increasing ability to accurately adjust one's mental model as a problem situation evolves. The purpose of an unfolding case study is to provide opportunities to observe and assess students' ability to change their mental model of a problem situation when they are presented with additional information that might expand the scope of the problem, confirm some hypothetical problem parameters but not others, or even conflict with their original conceptualization of the problem.

## Student Population:

I and my colleagues use 'unfolding case studies' to provide our students with a guided learning experience. A case that unfolds (presented to the student gradually) is a better model of how case information emerges in practice, and is optimal for training clinical reasoning. With new information evolving as the student thinks about the clinical judgments required in the case, they are required to make adjustments to their mental models of the clinical problems.

We teach this lesson to senior-level baccalaureate nursing students. Seniors have quire a bit of clinical knowledge and also enough clinical experience to realize that some cases are more complex than they initially appear. This teaching strategy is intended to capture the experience of the emergence of additional key clinical information about a case that occurs in practice and to prepare students for the need to rethink and adapt their mental model of the case. However, unfolding cases could and should be used for students at all levels, taking care to evolve the new case information as their clinical reasoning skills permit.

In our course and in this example the content area for the unfolding case is community health nursing, but any specialty area or subject matter can be used to create the case. This teaching strategy is appropriate whenever one is interested in guiding students' skills in mental models and assessing their ability to use them dynamically. One can teach this lesson to both individual students and student teams.

## Timing of Session:

We use this exercise at the end of the semester in our community health course. By that time, our students have read and discussed all of the material related to the topic and we have largely met our teaching objectives for presenting key community health content. This exercise is extremely useful for assessing our learning goals for the students. They have had time to mentally structure the new knowledge in their memory. The unfolding case tests their ability to retrieve and use this new knowledge in a novel case situation. As a result, requiring a written response to an unfolding case is a useful format for a final examination in a course. We describe the format for this use here

Unfolding cases can also be used more broadly in the course. For instance one could introduce this experience to the students at the start of the semester. They are not likely to be as accomplished in their ability to construct the optimal mental model of the community health problem, given their relative lack of content knowledge in this specialty area. But the introduction of this thinking experience early in the course allows them to learn the expectations we have for them by the time the semester closes. A comparison of the early unfolding case experience and the final end of course exercise would thus provide a pretest – posttest design that reflects learning in the area of the use of mental models as well as learning in the course content area.

**Materials:**

We have developed a format for our unfolding cases. Each consists of several consecutive "stages" that are revealed to students, one at a time. The first stage introduces the problem situation and provides enough information for the student to develop an initial mental model of the case. Subsequent stages provide additional information. As the case unfolds, the additional information provided might be highly relevant to the needed clinical judgment, only peripheral to the case, or even irrelevant to the clinical problems the case entails. An example of an unfolding case is included here (See Figure 1).

The difficult work for the instructor, of course, is designing the case and each of its stages well. Instructors may adopt published case studies or develop their own. Either way, the professor needs to think through each case as the students will later be doing. It is important to assure that they will be able to achieve useful mental models. Optimally these models assist them in efficiently synthesizing the new course content as well. Inclusion of irrelevant information at all stages is not a frivolous exercise. When this is well done, the case feels like an actual clinical reasoning experience. When students think aloud and share their emerging mental models this allows instructors to assess if students can differentiate significant from non-significant data. We organize this exercise by preparing all of the case materials in writing and distribute each new stage to students once they have completed thinking and discussing the previous stage. After reading each stage, students answer a set of questions designed to elicit aspects of their mental models. By asking the same question set after each stage and comparing answers across stages, changes in their mental models can be detected.

---

**The Unfolding Case**

**Stage 1**

You are a nurse at the State Health Department. On Wednesday morning, you receive a telephone call from a student at a nearby university who reports that he and his two roommates became ill with nausea, vomiting, and diarrhea after eating at a Chinese restaurant the night before. Two of the students recently returned from travel outside of the United States. None of the roommates have sought medical care and ask if they should skip their scheduled classes that day (all of them have an exam that afternoon). The students are not willing to give you their names or contact information.

**Stage 2**

Before the call is ended, you complete an *Illness Complaint Report* as required for all incoming calls. You consider whether or not to investigate further as you review the following information:

The roommates' ages range from 18 to 20.
Symptoms include: nausea, vomiting, diarrhea, fatigue (all 3 students); fever (1 student); headache (1 student).
None of the roommates report chills, bloody stool, abdominal cramps, muscle aches, or dizziness.
The students had dinner together at a local Chinese restaurant buffet the previous evening. They shared no other meals on the previous 2 days, although all of their meals were eaten at the university cafeteria.
Two of the roommates returned from a trip to Toronto, Canada, on Sunday evening.
Other than their current problem, they are in good health.

**Stage 3**

You decide to investigate further to establish facts about this case and to find out if others were also ill. First, you call the Chinese restaurant; however, you get no answer because the restaurant has not opened yet. You call the university's Student Health Center and learn that 18 students were seen yesterday for complaints of nausea, vomiting and diarrhea. They report that usually they see 1-2 cases like this per week. Finally, you call the local hospital Emergency Department. The Medical Director tells you he will check their records and get back with you later in the day.

---

Figure 1: Unfolding Case Study – Example Illness in a Community

In the community health nursing course, assessment focuses on students' responses to complex public health issues. We use the cases to help students explore these issues and possible solutions. There is a structure to our guidance in the case and examining each of these aspects helps students think a bit more about their reasoning process. This structure includes some reflection on *problem identification (PI), pattern recognition (PR), inferences (INF), hypotheses testing (HG)*, and *solution generation* (SG).

To guide mental model formation and adaptation, we repeatedly pose a list of questions after each stage of the unfolding case study. We ask the questions to help students analyze how their conceptualizations of the case are being developed, how information is being used when forming perceptions about the case, how they are using new information to affirm or dispute previous mental model conceptualizations, and how they are analyzing case data, drawing inferences and making explanations about possible interventions. The questions also help uncover underlying beliefs or assumptions being made about the causes of the problem(s). Answers to questions are compared across stages. Here is a brief guide of the repeated question format we use.

1) Based on what you know about this situation, what problem(s) should the clinician address? (PI)

2) What information did you use to identify each listed problem(s)? Why is the information relevant? (PR)

3) What do you think is causing the problem(s)? Why? (INF)

4) What additional information would you like to know about this case? Why? What problem(s) have you ruled out based on what you know now? Why? (HT)

5) What actions should the clinician consider taking? Why? (SG)

Figure 2 shows an example of two grids we have designed to capture the students' responses to these questions. Notice that the column order is slightly different (column 4 and 5) in the response grids than the question order above. This is done to emphasize that students should be seeking additional information to better inform their mental model.

***We ask students why at each stage***. This is important. In this case, asking why they are drawing specific inferences and making specific clinical judgments in column 3 and 4 potentially uncovers mistaken content knowledge about their synthesis of the community health content. Asking why in column 5 allows us to be sure that they are doing more than simply looking for information to confirm their initial mental model. We want to encourage them to continue to evolve their mental model through hypothesis generation and information seeking.

## COMMUNITY FOCUSED NURSING CASE STUDY – Stage 1

After reading Stage 1 of the Case Study, answer the following questions. When you are finished and ready to move to the next stage, turn in this page to your instructors and get Stage 2 materials.

| Column 1 | Column 2 | Column 3 | Column 4 | Column 5 |
|---|---|---|---|---|
| Based on what you know about this situation, what problem(s) should the nurse address? | What information did you use to identify each listed problem(s)? | What do you think is causing the problem(s)? Why? | What actions do you think the nurse should take? Why? | What additional information would you like to know about this situation? Why? |
| | | | | |
| | | | | |
| | | | | |
| | | | | |

## COMMUNITY FOCUSED NURSING CASE STUDY
### To be used with Stage 2 and additional Stages

After reading the new Stage of the Case Study, answer the following questions. When you are finished and ready to move to the next stage, please turn in this page and get the materials for the next Stage of this case.

| Column 1 | Column 2 | Column 3 | Column 4 | Column 5 |
|---|---|---|---|---|
| Based on what you know about this situation, what problem(s) should the nurse address? | What information did you use to identify each listed problem(s)? | What do you think is causing the problem(s)? Why? | What actions do you think the nurse should take? Why? | What additional information would you like to know about this situation? Why? |
| | | | | |
| | | | | |
| | | | | |
| | | | | |

What previously listed problem(s), if any, did you rule out based on what you know now? Why?

Figure 2: Two Grids for Entering Responses to the Unfolding Case

## Learning Outcomes Assessment

Assessment of learning achieved in this lesson can be focused on a variety of aspects. The repeated posed questions should be changed to emphasize the chosen area. For example, some possible outcomes that could be studied using this teaching strategy include: 1) how students perceive problems related to the situation and possible solutions that could be tried, 2) how well students can recall information about a case; 3) how students envision the outcome of a case if there is no intervention or if a certain specific action is taken; 4) how students construct their arguments about what is at issue in the case; or 5) how students assess the difficulty or risk associated with the case situation.

Depending on the level of the student and the intended learning outcome, it might be important for students to retain copies of their initial stage grids. Students thought that they would find it helpful to have a copy of each grid to help them remember what they had said previously about the case. Because we did not want them to alter their original answers, we allowed them to use a copy machine that was located outside the classroom to retain a copy of their earlier stage responses. However, not allowing students to make notes or copies of their work as they progress through the case forces an increased reliance on the mental model they have formed. It also requires students to rely more heavily on their recall of details of the problem situation, a more authentic test of actual clinical practice demands. We believe that the level of recall of details of the problem situation reflects level of expertise, with recall increasing as the person develops more sophisticated mental models of the domain.

## The Student Work Product:

Students enter their answers on a grid and complete a new grid for each stage of the case. Because we want students to think again about the case each time they are provided additional clinical information (at each stage), we ask students to submit each stage's response to the instructors before beginning the next stage. This way we can also use the data to assess their evolving mental model, because they have not added or erased responses to prior stages based on the new information. The final set of grids represents how the students' mental model evolved as new case information became available.

If team mental models are being evaluated, team members work together to discuss their impressions of the case and then come to a consensus as they complete the response grids. Only one set of grids is completed per team. Instructors may assign students to team member roles (e.g., recorder, leader) or let students determine this on their own.

**Evaluating Answers:**

All of us develop strategies for evaluating this type of work product. Here are some we have found to be useful and fair. After reading all students' work, we often subjectively compare students' answers, one to another, ranking them along a continuum of quality from low to high and assigning a score or pass/fail designation to each. We also typically compare student answers to an ideal referent. Scoring rubrics or guidelines should be developed that weight aspects of the students' work. For example, we assign higher and lower scores under criteria suggested in Figure 3.

The rubric can be used by students to evaluate their own or another student's grids, or by student teams in the same manner. The rubric should be shared in advance with the students as a effective way to set expectations about the exercise. The instructor's evaluation of the grids could be reviewed with each individual student or only with those who are struggling with clinical reasoning as a way to openly evaluate, praise and critique their clinical reasoning ability. In the case of students who are exceptionally weak in this area, objective evidence of this weakness proves highly useful for academic counseling.

When the students' responses are to be graded, you will need to explain your expectations fully before starting the exercise. Problem definition is a higher order thinking skill and as a result students are likely to be initially anxious about the exercise, and whether they will be able to get the 'right' answer. Case studies, however, usually have high appeal as a testing format once students begin the work. We begin by distributing the first stage of the case and page one of the grids. After students have read and responded to the first stage, they turn in their answers and receive the second stage of the case and page two of the grid. This continues until all stages of the case have been completed. We most often use three-stage unfolding cases in order to keep evaluation of answers for our large classes manageable. Notice that the grids for Stages 2 and above ask the additional question, "What previously listed problem(s), if any, did you rule out based on what you know now? Why?"

**Feedback from the Students:**

Students are generally positive about the experience, noting that they feel challenged by the cases. Comments include that the case studies are more like what they might encounter in the "real world" where decisions must often be made before all information is available. Some feel that getting up to turn in their answers and retrieve the next stage is somewhat disruptive to problem solving. This may not be an issue in smaller classes where the instructor can pick up/deliver materials to the students' desks after a signal of readiness to move on to the next stage. Another solution is to deliver the unfolding case on-line where students can move on once they have submitted responses to a previous stage. Students appreciate a general debriefing on the cases immediately following the exercise while the information is still fresh on their minds.

| Scores for Case Evaluation | |
|---|---|
| **Higher Scores** | **Evidence for grade or evaluation** |
| Identify critical problems early in the case (after initial case information) | List problem |
| Requests for additional information significant for clarify a problem or possible solution | List example |
| Correctly ruled out problem when refuting information was introduced | List example |
| **Lower Scores** | **Evidence for grade or evaluation** |
| Identify critical problems late in the case (after all information was available) | List problem |
| Requests for additional information that was irrelevant or would not contribute to problem clarification or solution | List example |
| Failed to rule out a problem when refuting information was introduced | List example |
| **Figure 3: Rubric for Evaluating the unfolding case** | |

## References

Azzarello, J. (2006). Assessing dynamic mental models: Unfolding case studies. *Nurse Educator*, 31 (1), 10-14.

Senge, P.M. *The fifth discipline: The art & practice of learning organizations.* New York: Doubleday, 1990.

# Roleplay Strategies for Critical Thinking in Psychiatric Mental Health

## Tim Blake

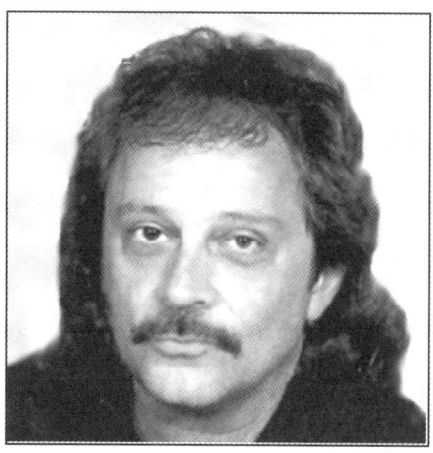

*Tim Blake is an Assistant Professor of Nursing at Ohio University, Zanesville, Ohio, USA. He and his colleagues have studied the differences in achieved learning outcomes stemming from traditional classroom teaching and on-line education. The cognitive-behavioral techniques of demonstration and behavioral modeling, roleplay, and providing feedback have long been known to be helpful in therapeutic interventions. Here Professor Blake uses roleplay to help students begin to better recognize and interact with patients with personality disorders. Consider using this same case scenario in a clinical conference as a way of working out how the staff will respond consistently and therapeutically to particularly difficult patients. During the role play all students are engaged in higher order thinking processes to interpret, analyze and draw an inference on the nature of the personality disorder being manifested by the 'patient.'*

## Class Session and students

I teach this class to second year associate degree nursing students as part of an introductory psychiatric – mental health nursing course. The course is part of their preparation for caring for patients with psychiatric disorders. They have already completed an introductory psychology course as a prerequisite to this course, and at the end of this year of study, students will sit for the certification examination to practice as a registered nurse.

## The Goal of the class session

For most students, personality disorders are a somewhat difficult group of psychiatric disorders to understand, let alone recognize. My goal for this lesson is to help the students to understand and begin to recognize three of the more common personality disorders they may encounter in the health care setting.

'Recognizing' the disorder implies having the disposition to observe and interpret verbalizations and behaviors with a view to analyzing their pattern and implications, drawing a correct inference about the psychiatric disorder being expressed. These are all cognitive behaviors and habits of mind that involve critical thinking. I stress that recognition of personality disorders will assist them in maintaining a working relationship with the patient, whether they are working with them in the psychiatric unit, the clinic, or in a community setting. Role play is an excellent means of demonstrating the behaviors of such disorders. For additional discussions of roleplay as a strategy for elaborating a problem focused thinking process, see the paper by Dalrymple and colleagues (2007) at the University of Southern California School of Dentistry. They discuss the use of roleplay as integral to problem based learning.

**Actual material used for the class session**

Any psychiatric textbook that deals well with personality disorders would be appropriate. I particularly favor those texts that take a critical thinking approach to presenting the content and include critical thinking questions at the chapter end or throughout the text. Students are expected to prepare for class by reading about and thinking about each disorder.

**Learning Objectives and the critical thinking involved**

After participating in this lesson, students will be able to:

- Determine the type of personality disorder that is being portrayed in the role play based upon student comparisons with assigned readings. (analysis and inference).
- Analyze their insights from the roleplay exercise and determine the behavioral, affective, cognitive, and socio-cultural characteristics portrayed by the client who has one of three personality disorders. (interpretation and analysis).
- Compare and contrast the causative theories underlying personality disorders.
- Describe specific nursing interventions that are appropriate for the client portrayed in the role play, along with rationale for the interventions (analysis and explanation).
- Discuss personal reactions to the character portrayed in the role play and their potential effect on the nurse – client relationship. (Analysis, interpretation and explanation, as well as the critical thinking disposition of truth-seeking).
-

## How I teach this lesson

Lessons that involve roleplay exercises as a way of better engaging the real problems presented in a situation require some thoughtful choices. What roles are required if the learning objects are to be met? Who should play each of the roles? In an exercise where the goal is to have the health care team identify the health problem involved or think through the implications of a particular illness condition, the instructor will often want to play the role of the patient and carefully evolve what the students come to know about the patient's condition. If the goal is rather to sensitize providers or student providers to the problems associated with the illness condition, or to difficulties associated with seeking health care, it works best to have them act the role of the patient.

In this role play, my learning goals involve the students' recognition of the disorder, so I play the part of a patient who has been admitted to the hospital. I ask one student to volunteer to be the "nurse" who provides care for me for that day. This student is then responsible for completing an assessment on me, the patient, focusing on asking me questions that might help them to determine what type of personality disorder she or he is dealing with. During the interview to follow, I try to create the feeling that we are really a nurse and patient in an intake assessment so that the student will think well and ask appropriate questions.

The rest of the class also has a responsibility. They are the "peanut gallery," and they play the part of the nurse's "mind." In this role, they are allowed to prompt the nurse by asking questions that can help in the nurse's evaluation. This way everyone stays engaged in the exercise, and has an opportunity and the responsibility to take part in the evaluation of the client. If the session gets off track, I have the option to jump out of role and become the professor again, but this is rarely necessary. It's more common that someone from the peanut gallery offers a question in what would otherwise be an awkward silence if only one student were on the hot spot conducting the interview. Generally speaking, the majority of the class takes part in the assessment, asking questions relevant to each part of the patient's cognitive, behavioral, affective, and socio-cultural domains.

So in the actual roleplay, for example, I specifically take on the role of a person with an antisocial personality. To prepare for the roleplay, I develop a specific patient history before the lesson. This preparation assures that my roleplay will be as authentic a portrayal as possible. The history of the patient that I have in mind for this lesson is shown in Figure 1.

88  Critical Thinking and Clinical Reasoning in the Health Sciences: A Teaching Anthology

> **Social History for this patient:**
>
> The patient goes by the name of Roy. He grew up in a home where the father was an alcoholic. The father was physically abusive to Roy's mother, Roy, and his sister. When Roy was 14 years old, his father killed his mother in a fit of rage, and Roy was forced to go live with relatives. His sister had been sexually abused for years by the father. As a teenager, she would be committed to a state mental facility where she has remained. Roy has had no contact with her or his father.
>
> Roy also has a history of heavy drinking and drug abuse (marijuana), and generally uses both on a daily basis. He has done most other drugs when he has the opportunity. He is not currently married, and lived with a number of women in the past. These relationships usually don't work out because "they just don't listen very well." He has no problem "beating a woman around" to knock them into shape or to get them to listen, adding "this is my world and they're just livin' in it."
>
> Roy also has a history of prison time for manslaughter and grand theft, but denies any responsibility for any of his actions, stating that it is generally someone else's fault. When confronted with any of this behavior, he demonstrates no remorse for his past behaviors or for infringing on the rights of others.

**Figure 1: Roleplaying 'Roy'**

This case history is not known to the student nurse at the time when the interview begins. If the nurse (and the other students) ask the right questions, they are able to elicit all of this information from "Roy." The students do have information about Roy's admission to the Unit (Figure 2).

> Roy was admitted to the hospital after an incident that occurred at work where he had an altercation with another employee. He threatened to kill the employee by cutting his throat. The employee told the supervisor, who called Roy into his office. Roy admitted that he had indeed "promised" to cut the man's throat because he didn't like him. Roy's supervisor told him that if he hoped to keep his job, he must seek help immediately or he would be fired. Because he needed the job, Roy went to the hospital and reported that he was homicidal. Thus, he was admitted to the psychiatric unit for treatment.

**Figure 2: Roy's Admission History**

I roleplay 'Roy' with enough passion to draw the student nurse and the group into the dialogue, and they successfully come up with appropriate questions. I generally try to make "Roy" as obnoxious as possible because this is what psychiatric nurses are likely to encounter! Sometime the interviewer struggles but when this occurs they have the assistance of the class to help guide them along. This guidance usually prompts them in the right direction.

After about 15 minutes, I bring the patient interview to a close and ask the group if they can identify my diagnosis along with evidence to back up their claim (analyze, infer and explain). The evidence for their proposed diagnosis must be based on the readings that they've done and this helps them to put it all together. This session is a think aloud where everyone works to recall what was said by Roy and to connect it to what is known about the disorders we are studying. In this case the correct diagnosis is 'antisocial disorder.' In the event that you are unfamiliar with this disorder, Table 1 shows the cues in the roleplay that students should identify as significant when they make the clinical judgment that Roy has antisocial disorder,

---

**Table 1: Key Characteristics of Antisocial Disorder**

**Social history:**

- Drug and alcohol abuse (common with these individuals)
- Childhood home that was quite chaotic and dysfunctional
- Victim of violence
- Numerous relationships with women which don't seem to last (because the women don't "seem to listen" to him, and meet his every need)

**Personality characteristics:**

- Egocentricism: Antisocial personalities see themselves at the center of their universe. Roy shows this attribute when he says "this is my world and they're just livin' in it."
- Lack of remorse for past behavior: This type of client is unable to empathize with others, and is therefore unable to understand how his actions affect them.

**Behaviors:**

- Prone to violent behavior (the likely result of his father's demonstrated violence)
- Limited problem solving skills. When Roy is faced with a conflict involving others, he solves it by simply infringing upon the rights of others, a hallmark of antisocial personalities.

---

After we have completed the discussion of the case, I ask the group to evaluate the performance of the student nurse who "assessed" the patient in the role play. Did the student respond in a therapeutic manner? While it is not a specific learning objective of this course, developing the "art" of therapeutic communication is a program level learning objective that is addressed here. Varcarolis, (2006) put it very succinctly when saying that therapeutic communication provides the client with the opportunity to feel understood and comfortable, to identify and explore the problem they are having with significant others, to explore positive coping methods and to experience a satisfying therapeutic relationship.

I also ask myself, "Did the students use other appropriate interventions that had been previously explored during class? An example of evidence that students were asking therapeutic questions might be if they had asked Roy "Can you tell me more about this problem?" or "Can you describe that feeling in more detail?" A therapeutic statement might seek clarification. For example, "I'm not certain I'm following what you're saying. Can you tell me more?" Or "What would you say is the main point of what you have just said?" One example of a non-therapeutic statement would be giving advice to patients. For example "You should just get out of that relationship now!" Another common mistake which can obstruct communication is giving approval to a client. For example "You look great today, Mrs. Smith." Such an innocent statement can imply to the client that she looked terrible prior to today.

In debriefing the group exercise, there are many more opportunities to engage the group in critical thinking as they evaluate their group roleplay. In this case, being sure to ask for the reasons why they are making their critical comments pushes them to reanalyze the exercise and explain the reasons why they have either complimented or criticized the interviewer's work.

During the remaining class period, we continue to discuss theory relevant to the antisocial personality as well as other the personality disorders. We also discuss appropriate nursing interventions for dealing with such difficult patients and how they could have been applied to "Roy." I take some time to elicit student feedback on their immediate reactions to the role play.

### Student feedback on the roleplay exercise

I can see that every student in the class is absolutely engaged in the roleplay process. It's as if they can't wait to see what's going to transpire next. And, because they are all actually part of the process, it's as though each of them has more of a vested interest in the outcome of the interview. After all, each of them is free to ask a question that they feel is appropriate. I've found that when I allow Roy to be quite obnoxious, it draws students right into the situation. For instance, I can provoke students into losing sight of their clinical role and arguing with Roy, particularly when it comes to his views on abusing women. I've even had students yell at Roy (obviously, not a therapeutic communication!) But this class session is the place to provoke this type of reaction if it is going to occur, so that students can learn how to control these responses in this safe student environment.

Here is one definite opportunity to examine personal reactions to the patient in a truth-seeking way. Asking ourselves hard questions about why we find it difficult to work therapeutically with Roy is an important part of the training of the psychiatric health professional. The debriefing the roleplay offers the entire group the opportunity to study the interaction from a perspective of analyzing the non-therapeutic exchange and drawing inferences about why it was difficult to maintain a professional and therapeutic relationship with Roy. If I am successful with the roleplay exercise, all have gained some insight into how they will work with the real 'Roy' when they meet him in the clinical environment.

Typically 35-40% of the students specifically mention this roleplay exercise in their comments about the course when they complete course evaluations at the end of the quarter. The mention how much they enjoyed and learned from the role play and that would like to see more of this type of case exercise. One could use this strategy more than once in a course with the goal of carrying out a real time clinical evaluation of a patient and working on their therapeutic communication skills.

## Evaluation of Student Learning Objectives

Formal evaluation of the students' completion of the class objectives comes through examination questions. I use multiple choice questions to evaluate the knowledge that students have gained on personality disorders. I choose questions where there is only one correct answer, and where it can be explained why all of the other answer choices are incorrect. If your class is not too large to grade open format questions, asking students to explain why wrong answers are wrong practices them in the critical thinking skill of explanation and provides evidence that they identify the correct answer for the correct reason.

## References

Blake, T. (Epub 2005, 2006). Journaling as an Active Learning Technique. *International Journal of Nursing Education Scholarship*, 2 (1), Article 7, Apr.15th.

Blake, T., Jones, S., & Sweet, S. (2006). Adult Learning: A comparison of traditional vs. on-line methods of delivery. *AURCO Journal.* vol. 12.

Dalrymple, K.R., Wuenschell, C., Rosenblum, A., Paine, M., Crowe, D., von Bergmann, H.C., Wong, S., Bradford, M.S., & Schuler, C.F. (2007). PBL core skills faculty development workshop 1: An experiential exercise with the PBL process. *Journal of Dental Education*, 71(2), 249-59.

Henderson, D., Sealover, P., Sharrer, V., Fusner, S., Jones, S., Sweet, S., & Blake, T. (2006). Nursing EDGE: Evaluating delegation guidelines in education. *International Journal of Nursing Education Scholarship*, 3 (1), E-publication, March 16, 2006.

Varcarolis, E. *Foundations of mental health nursing: A clinical approach,* 5$^{th}$ Ed. New York, NY: Saunders, 2006.

# Keeping a Journal of Reflections on Learning

## *Anna Chur-Hansen*

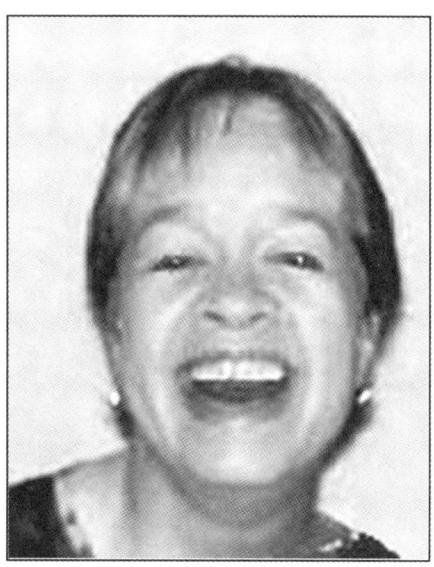

*Dr Anna Chur-Hansen is currently Acting Head, in the Discipline of Psychiatry at the Royal Adelaide Hospital, University of Adelaide, South Australia. She is a Registered Psychologist, advocating for interdisciplinary approaches to health care and the teaching of health care professionals, and holds a Ph.D. from the University of Adelaide in Medical Education. She chairs the Australian Psychological Society's College of Health Psychologists (South Australian Branch) and is a Senior Advisor to the United States Association of Psychologists in Academic Health Centres Board of Directors. Her research on teaching and learning in the health professions and health psychology focuses on the patient's perceptions of their learning experiences.*

*In this chapter Dr. Chur-Hansen talks eloquently about a portfolio journal exercise she includes as a mechanism of course evaluation and learning assessment in the courses she teaches to health science students at the University of Adelaide. Here the term 'portfolio' is used to refer to a formative self-evaluation tool that encourages reflective evaluation of learning from the student's perspective. (Other uses of the term refer to the collection of a 'showcase portfolio' where students collect only their best work and use it for job placement, or 'assessment portfolios' where an objective sampling of student work products are collected for the purpose of curriculum or program level assessment).*

*This thoughtful exercise emphasizes the practice of analysis, inference, and evaluation. It also calls upon students to be fair-minded in their critique, training the critical thinking dispositions of truth-seeking and open-mindedness. Reflective journaling is used with careful guidance to developing the important skill of metacognitive reflection summed up by one of the journaling directions:*

*"Consider why you think so."* This habit of mind is at the heart of competent clinical reasoning at every level of expertise. Other helpful theoretical and research papers by Dr. Chur-Hansen are included in the reference list at the end of the chapter.

## Background and Context

It is widely accepted that knowledge about health should be based on interdisciplinary collaboration. There are several reasons for this: first, health care providers work in teams; second, both the aetiology and treatment of many conditions, including high prevalence chronic illnesses such as diabetes and hypertension are becoming increasingly multimodal; third, it is well recognised that holistic approaches to health and health care are desirable over the reductionist approaches of the recent past; and fourth, an interdisciplinary approach to medical and psychological research is now encouraged - perhaps expected - by institutions and granting bodies.

Medical, psychology and health sciences students learn together in two courses offered at the University of Adelaide, the first year course of "Person, Culture and Medicine" (referred to hereafter as PCM), and the second year course that follows, "Emotion, Culture and Medicine" (ECM). In these courses the topics of food and eating, sex and relationships, pain and death, and human emotional states in health and illness are examined from psychological, cultural and physical anthropological and neurobiological perspectives. Representatives from each discipline contribute to teaching sessions. The pedagogical underpinning of this approach is that health issues are best understood by combining knowledge from different disciplines. For this to occur, people from these seemingly disparate disciplines must work together with understanding and respect. To the best of my knowledge this course is unique in its aims, these being: the facilitation of interdisciplinary approaches to a number of aspects of human variation as they occur throughout the life-cycle; an appreciation that psychology, cultural anthropology, physical anthropology and neurobiology are complementary disciplines, and that sometimes they intersect; and an understanding of the complexity of and variation in human responses to major life events.

## Rationale behind the journal

There is a strong movement in the health professions, and particularly in nursing and in medicine, towards fostering "reflective practice" (Schon, 1987). There is also a movement, again primarily in medicine, toward the use of portfolios for teaching and learning. Both of these approaches are extremely valuable for lifelong learning and the facilitation of critical thinking. Thus, students in PCM and ECM are required to maintain a reflective portfolio – in other words, a journal, or diary – of their thoughts and experiences in relation to their studies. They are encouraged to make links to their wider learning experiences at university. As partners in the teaching and learning process, the portfolio is one vehicle for them to express their satisfaction or constructive criticisms about the course.

## Learning objectives of the exercise

Based on the rationale of the reflective portfolio, it aims to achieve the following learning objectives:

(a) Introduction to the concept of maintaining a journal in which thoughts about teaching and learning experiences in class are recorded.

(b) Development of critical reflection skills about the course and one's own abilities, including strengths and weaknesses in relation to course requirements, and course aims and objectives.

(c) Development of evaluative reasoning skills in providing constructive criticism to the course coordinator through writing in the journal.

(d) An understanding that this exercise and these skills may be useful outside the class context – for example, in other courses, in other professional arenas.

In working toward the achievement of objectives 'b' and 'c' the emphasis is on practice the critical thinking skills of analysis, inference and evaluation. I also expect a fair-minded and constructive approach to the critical reflection and evaluative critique of the course.

## What is expected from class participants?

In the medical education literature there are many examples of "failures" when using journals and portfolios. Driessen and colleagues (2005) have outlined the conditions under which portfolios are most likely to succeed in helping students to learn. These conditions, which have been followed in PCM and ECM, are (1) the provision of formative feedback; (2) the provision of clear guidelines; (3) latitude for the student to write freely if they wish; (4) exposure to experiences worth writing about; and (5) the award of a pass or fail grade. I use all of these suggestions in the design of this portfolio exercise.

**Instructions for the Journal Exercise**

- There must be a minimum of 12 entries in the journal in order to achieve a satisfactory grade (one for each class). There is no maximum limit of entries, nor is there a minimum or maximum length requirement.
- The portfolio can be presented in any way you wish – written in an exercise book, or typed onto separate, stapled sheets.
- Each entry must be dated.
    - You can reflect upon your experience in the course in any ways you feel are appropriate. Typical entries may revolve around what you are learning, looking back upon it, thinking through plans for assessment tasks, considering where your knowledge is lacking, reflecting upon emotional reactions to material in the course, the ways in which you are being taught, how you feel about your learning experiences and so on.
    - You may also like to think through whether the course is achieving its stated aims and objectives. For example, have some of your ideas and beliefs been challenged? How do you feel about that? Do you think it is useful to learn alongside students from other disciplines or not? Consider why you think so.
- In assessing portfolios, higher grades will be awarded to students who show an ability to reflect in an open and honest way that fosters insight into their learning. Credit will be given for students who show development over the period of the portfolio.
- Some things are not appropriate for portfolios, for example: personally insulting remarks about classmates or teachers, and sexist or racist reflections.
- However, negative feelings, criticisms about the teaching or the course, disappointment about the experience and so on are acceptable and indeed, can be powerful in helping you to achieve an insight into yourself and how you deal with such things. For example, think through why you feel unhappy, and what you might be able to do to constructively manage the issue. If you are not sure how to word such reflections, Dr Chur-Hansen will help you with this during a formative feedback session.

**Figure 1**

At the Orientation Class (the very first class meeting) students are advised that part of the assessment requirement for the course will involve keeping a reflective portfolio, which contributes 10% toward the final, summative grade. The rationale behind asking students to maintain a reflective journal, and what is expected, is discussed. In explaining the purpose of the portfolio, students hear about the literature's evidence for the value of reflection in learning and in clinical practice. They also learn that reflection is a skill, and needs to be worked upon throughout the course and beyond. Figure 1 displays the instructions I give to students for this exercise.

Students are required to receive formative feedback at least once (but as many times as they wish) on their portfolio. This is important, since for almost all students in the courses it is the first time that they have been asked to keep a reflective journal. For most, it is the first time that they have been asked to step away from learning factual material, and to instead consider the process of learning itself. It is also the first time they may have been asked to take some responsibility for the provision of formative feedback to their teachers, as adult learners. These are sophisticated expectations that require guidance.

In addition to adding metacognitive reflection about their learning process, this journaling exercise requests that they use critical thinking skills to produce their journal entries: analyzing exactly what they see as evidence of learning; explaining how they interpret the learning experience; analyzing their emotional responses to course content; drawing inferences as to the appropriateness of these responses; comparing expected learning goals and objectives with actual learning outcomes; interpreting and evaluating the instructor's teaching methods. All of these call for the practice of critical thinking skills.

**Evaluating the Portfolios**

You can see that I have provided to the students my evaluation criteria embedded in Figure 1. Figure 2 pulls these out for easier consideration. The guidelines communicate to students that I value open and honest reflection that fosters insight into their learning and growth in the skills of critical reflection over time. I encourage a thoughtful critique of the course in terms of the learning experiences they are having, and offer to help them develop the critique skills needed for a thoughtful discussion of how they are measuring progress toward and barriers to learning. I also make it clear that fair-minded analysis and evaluation is what is needed, and not ad hominem arguments or groundless prejudicial attacks.

---
**Criteria for Evaluating the Portfolios**

12 dated journal entries at minimum

Reflections on many of the following:

- Feelings and emotional reactions: to course content, analysing their meaning and appropriateness
- Learning in the course and continuing knowledge gaps
- The accomplishment of class assessment tasks
- Observations their response to varying teaching modalities
- Reflections of the achievement of the courses' stated aims and objectives
- Reflections on the experience of having ideas and beliefs challenged
- Reflections on being taught in a multidisciplinary learning environment
---

Figure 2

## Student responses and feedback

The portfolios are a challenge to students. The medical students in the class have a basic familiarity with the concept, but the portfolios they keep for their medical studies are concerned with their reflections around interactions with patients and clinical questions. They do not reflect on a deep level about their own learning and learning processes. For the psychology and health sciences students, the concept of a portfolio that documents their thoughts and emotional reactions is quite alien. The portfolio for PCM and ECM is solely concerned with reflections about learning and teaching matters. None of the students have ever had to think about the ways in which they are learning new material, how material links with prior knowledge, how the delivery of the course helps or hampers their individual learning styles and needs, or to put themselves in the shoes of their teacher – that is, what they think about the educational approaches being used and the material presented.

For those who master the skill of reflection about theio r own learning process the benefit is immediate and lasting. *However, the portfolio has not always facilitated student learning.* There is a tendency for some students to simply summarize the class content, rather than demonstrate true critical reflection, upon which assessment of the portfolio is based. These students become frustrated, seeing the exercise as a waste of time. Most, however, enjoy the exercise and learn a great deal from it. To encourage engagement in this task in future PCM and ECM classes I intend to provide students with examples of thoughtful, reflective portfolio entries, something that I have not yet done.

The portfolio has definitely been an invaluable insight for me into students' thoughts and needs. It has most definitely helped me to understand why difficulties in learning arise, and gives me ideas on how to address these. Because I see the portfolio during formative feedback sessions, I am able to act on concerns during the course, not simply wait until the next group of students has commenced the year.

The following are excerpts from students' journals, illustrating the benefits for them:

> "It took me a while to get into this reflective journal, as I wasn't entirely sure it would be a useful exercise, however after a few weeks I started to enjoy writing about particular topics and discussions that I had found the most interesting. Often it was only passing comments or brief stories or explanations that caught my attention and interest, and it was good to be able to expand and reflect on those issues in this journal after the class" (PCM Year 1)

> "I've been finding the journal a really useful tool to nut out my ideas for the essays, and relate the questions to what we learn in class – but without even consciously meaning to. In PCM I was a bit reserved about the journal at first, and was skeptical about how effective it would really be in assisting me with my learning, but I have no doubts now. It's a shame that they don't make us do this in any of our other courses" (ECM Year 2)

> "I realise that I am one of those students who does not participate in discussions within the class. The reason why, I believe, is because I feel like most of the other students in the class . . . are more comfortable, knowledgeable and opinionated concerning the subjects in this course than I am. Writing this, I have just had a realisation – the purpose of this portfolio is to force us to bring things like this to our own attention. I will try and work on my participation from now on." (ECM Year 2)

## References

Chur-Hansen, A. (2001). Self-evaluation of medical communication skills. *Higher Education Research and Development*, 20, 71-79.
Chur-Hansen, A. & Koopowitz, L. (2005) The role of formative feedback in teaching undergraduate psychiatry. *Academic Psychiatry,* 29, 66-68.
Chur-Hansen, A., Parker, D., Henneberg, M. & Barrett, R. (2006). Interdisciplinary electives in the humanities for students of medicine, health sciences and psychology: suggestions and implications. *Focus on Health Professional Education*, 8, 32-39.

Driessen, E.W., van Tartwick, J., Overeem, K., Vermunt, J.D. & van der Vleuten, C.P. (2005). Conditions for successful reflective use of portfolios in undergraduate medical education. *Medical Education*, 39, 1230-1235.

Schon, D.A. *Educating the reflective practitioner: Toward a new design for teaching and learning in the professions.* San Francisco, Jossey-Bass, 1987.

Winefield, H.R. & Chur-Hansen, A. (2004). Integrating psychologists into primary mental health care in Australia. *Families, Systems and Health*, 22, 294-305.

Winefield, H.R. & Chur-Hansen, A.Working with a multi-disciplinary staff. In L.M. Cohen, D.E. McChargue & F.L. Collins (Eds). *The Health Psychology Handbook: Practical Issues for the Behavioral Medicine Specialist,* (pp. 28-41). Thousand Oaks, CA: Sage, 2003.

# Teachable Moments in Clinical Practice: Promoting Clinical Judgment Skills

## *Margot Thomas*

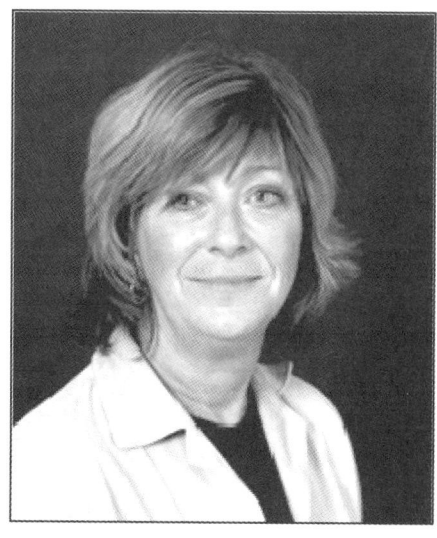

*Margot Thomas is an advanced practice nurse (APN) in the Pediatric Intensive Care Unit at Children's Hospital of Eastern Ontario, in Ottawa, Canada. As a critical care APN, she is directly involved in continuing professional development and competency acquisition of staff nurses caring for infants, children, and youth experiencing life threatening illnesses. She seeks to improve clinical judgment by focusing on the recognition of cues used by clinicians to make diagnostic inferences. Although this process requires the iterative use of the full range of critical thinking skills, Ms. Thomas centers this lesson on the practice of two of these skills: interpretation and explanation.*

*Others have tried to build the critical thinking skill of interpretation by asking students to continue to ponder a seemingly transparent situation until they uncover more subtle details that were previously unnoticed but prove to be highly significant. Here Ms. Thomas applies the idea of 'seizing a teachable moment,' a moment when the clinician is making a difficult decision. In the midst of the teachable moment, when asked "Why do you think that?" or "Why did you decide to do that?" the critical thinking task turns to talking aloud about the clinical reasoning process and explaining the clinical judgment. The idea is to capture a near to real time decision process. The result is likely to increase the habit of more closely monitoring the quality of one's own thinking (metacognition). This chapter is an interesting blend of phenomenology and cognitive theory. We think you will find this discussion helpful for identifying teachable moments in your own work and practice settings, and ways to incorporate this idea into your teaching of clinical reasoning.*

## Background

My focus as an APN is to assist staff nurses to acquire and maintain the competence and confidence necessary to provide safe patient care and to effectively participate as a full partner in the multidisciplinary health care team caring for patients and their families. This example focuses on the 'teachable moments' (Benner, Hooper-Kyriakidis & Stanndard, 1999; Rashotte & Thomas, 2002) that occur in the clinical setting where I have the opportunity to facilitate experiential learning, reflective practice (Schon, 1987), and transformative learning (Cranton, 1996; Cranton & Carusetta, 2004) in other members of my health care team. Teachable moments are occasions that spontaneously arise out of a 'ready-to-hand' clinical situation in which a practice question, concern, doubt, or uncertainty suddenly surfaces.

Usually teachable moments occur as short conversations at the bedside. They rarely last more than 15 minutes. Often the focus of the moment is to identify how best to proceed, or how to make the right or best decision in "this case." The term 'naturalistic decision' has been used to describe this type of real life decision, where there are high stakes consequences and where there is significant uncertainty (Zambok, & Klein, 1997). Nearly all clinical problems that present novel circumstances are of this type.

*My task as a clinical teacher is to seize or even create a teachable moment* where I can assist other clinicians or student clinicians to examine and refine or disconfirm and revise the assumptions or expectations they hold about what will occur in response to their actions. Although there is much value to staff development opportunities that are structured seminars, teachable moments most often occur when the teacher (e.g., advanced practice nurse, nurse educator, preceptor, senior resident, clinical instructor) connects with the clinician or health care team member at the bedside in response to their recognition of a patient problem and their own learning needs.

There are two kinds of situations where I try to seize the teachable moment. The first is when the patient assignment challenges the clinician's or student clinician's clinical expertise. One example is the situation that occurs when a nurse cares for an infant requiring high frequency oscillation for severe respiratory failure for the first time. The second is a bedside request for assistance with some 'needed' clinical intervention. In this chapter the example is a staff nurse's request for assistance from the advanced practice nurse. Help is needed to do endotracheal tube suctioning, and this brings an opportunity for a teachable moment when the staff nurse is likely to be open to learning about their reasoning process.

In essence, teachable moments are opportunities to critically and reflectively think out loud, thus making critical thinking both conscious and visible. Svenson (1989) described the value of thinking aloud as a way of externalizing one's thinking process so that it can be observed and evaluated by oneself and by others. When this is done well, the thinker has the potential to move theoretical and/or experiential knowing into a conscious, reflected upon, and articulated knowing-in-action.

## My goals for this learning opportunity

In the following example, my goal during the teachable moment is to focus on helping the novice staff nurse (learner) make linkages between her or his theoretical knowledge about mechanically ventilated infants (specifically the endotracheal tube suctioning procedure) and the specific decisions and actions needed to be carried out for this patient in this situation. The purpose of the interaction between learner and teacher is to draw forth the complexity of the real clinical situation, including the context and the unique attributes of this particular patient in real time - all of which cannot be learned in a didactic session. I also seek to keep the learner connected to multiple ways of knowing about the best course of action in this case. My interaction with the nurse during the teachable moment is intended to support the nurse in the development of a sense of knowing *this* particular patient, *this* type of patient, and *this* practice environment through this co-created, reflecting-in-action activity. Analysis of the unique aspects of this case makes it a worthy exemplar, and an explanation of why planned interventions are appropriate.

I have summarized my theoretical basis for how to guide a teachable moment with a particular focus on the skilled performance of endotracheal tube suctioning using a model of clinical judgment first proposed by Thomas & Fothergill-Bourbonnais (2005). Guiding the discussion about endotracheal suctioning using this model facilitates meeting a number of learning objectives (listed below). After each of the following learning objectives, I've also included mention of the critical thinking skill that is being practiced by the thinking process involved as they are briefly referred to in the APA Delphi Report.

## Learning objectives

Through guided conversation, the learner who participates in a teachable moment related to endotracheal tube suctioning will be able to:

- Articulate the patient cues (visual, auditory, tactile) to which they are attending in this patient/this type of patient/ this practice environment) they recognized as indicating a need for endotracheal tube suctioning; (interpretation)

- Discuss why they considered the cues recognized as important and relevant to the judgment, considering the general and the particular (weighing the evidence); (analysis and explanation)

- Consider alternative cues that might be relevant (although perhaps not present) to making the judgment to suction (analysis and inference);

- Describe the ways in which they corroborated the significance of those impressions with others or with practical knowledge (explanation); and

- Evaluate the quality of the judgment to suction in response to the cues recognized in the patient and in the clinical context (analysis and self-regulation, also known as metacognitive self-critique).

I also evaluate the quality of the nurses' technique in suctioning the child, and if this is not a high standard of care, I move to teaching the suctioning skills themselves.

**My work before the teachable moment**

In order to be able to connect with clinicians, and most particularly staff nurses, to assist them in developing the practical knowledge essential in a clinical context, I must understand the patients and their health care needs in the unit. It is the patients' needs associated with the clinician's learning gap that determines the focus and timing of a teachable moment. I often find the opportunity for these learning sessions by attending the daily health care team rounds in the Pediatric Intensive Care Unit, listening attentively to what clinicians say in order to assess their knowledge and understanding of the patients' clinical situations.

As a clinical expert, I come to this situation to assess the depth and breadth of the clinician's knowledge and understanding of this situation in order to identify any areas into which I can bring evidence to support or add to the reasoning that supports the clinician's practices. In addition, the teachable moment is an opportunity to engage the clinician in a discussion that identifies different ways of thinking about what is happening in this particular patient context and how it relates to this type of patient in general.

## Teaching the Teachable Moment

When I note that a clinician has been given an assignment that appears to challenge their expertise level, or potentially present them with novel patient care situations, I recognize the potential opportunity for a teachable moment. For instance, if I observe that a nurse has been given an assignment to care for an infant with severe respiratory failure for the first time, I make of point of coming back to talk with that nurse to both act as a resource and also to engage the nurse in a teachable moment about procedures that the nurse may need to perform for this child. For example, I might initially ask the nurse who is new to performing endotracheal tube suctioning, "Tell me about your patient today. How does the patient respond to being suctioned?" Or I might ask, "So what made you decide that the baby needed to be suctioned?" I've noticed that rather than listing the cues that they observed in the infant that they are suctioning, they will more often quickly recite the cues that are identified in the practice guidelines for suctioning. In this case they may say, "coughing, visible secretions, desaturations."

However, when I ask them to think aloud and tell me the story about what other cues they recognized in *this* patient, they may reveal other cues previously hidden from their immediate awareness. This storytelling becomes an opening to explore with the nurse other auditory, visual, and tactile cues that had also indicated this infant's need for suctioning. They might talk about the baby's restless behavior, grimacing, the pattern of the baby's breathing, tugging movements of the baby's shoulders, or the sensation of secretions felt when the nurse laid her/his hand on the baby's chest. The conversation becomes a chance for the nurse to reflect on this longer list of cues that they have now identified, and to more carefully analyze the meaning of these cues in context. Together the cues represent a pattern that the nurse comes to know as one where suctioning might be needed.

Weighing the evidence should be an important step in determining the timing and method of endotracheal tube suctioning. "When to suction?" may be a novel problem for new nurses. When I see that the nurse does have a knowledge gap and could benefit by analyzing their clinical judgment to suction the patient, I extend the conversation to discuss the specifics of the patient and clinical situation as a way of bringing forth how *knowing this patient* (how this baby responds to endotracheal tube suctioning) and *knowing this type of patient* (how babies in severe respiratory failure can develop complications from endotracheal tube suctioning) is relevant to the judgment of whether and/or when to suction. For example, I might ask the nurse to consider the significance of the cues recognized in this baby in relation to other pathophysiological conditions that may be relevant to the baby. This might be done by asking the nurse to identify situations when the judgment to suction might need to be reconsidered, or when collaboration with respiratory therapists might be indicated, such as when pulmonary hypertensive crises or severe bradycardic events can result.

I might also ask them to consider what other contextual factors influenced their decision-making to suction. This begins a thinking process where the nurse should be able to identify the evidence that supports their practice decision. And I am looking for particular responses that I can see to be relevant, such as the availability of backup support or the presence of family members. When they do provide appropriate comments, the ones I already had in mind or others I can see are relevant, I model the responsibility to be evidence based by offering additional explanation for why these are appropriate and important influences. If they fail to provide an adequate response, I suggest some relevant considerations and then listen as they integrate this information into their own thinking process.

When appropriate, I will stay at the bedside while the nurse performs endotracheal tube suctioning, purposefully observing for specific behaviors that the nurse implements as means of protecting the patient from the potential complications of endotracheal tube suctioning. Once the suctioning is completed, I ask the question, "When you were suctioning your patient, what was going through your mind?" as a way of helping the nurse reflect on her/his actions. Usually, the staff new to suctioning ventilated critically infants will respond with answers indicating a focus on information obtained from monitor equipment (e.g., heart rate, blood pressure, and oxygen saturations) and the effectiveness of suctioning (e.g., amount and color of the secretions obtained). This then becomes another opportunity to invite the nurse to consider other cues gathered and considered by expert pediatric critical care nurses (e.g., the sounds of secretions during the manual ventilation process, or resistance felt when the suction catheter is passed through the endotracheal tube), as well as other aspects of safe suctioning practice. This same approach to the teachable moment can be adapted to any other area of expertise in regard to excellent practice. In this pediatric unit other areas would include ways to reduce patient's distress, monitoring the number of suction passes, or protecting of the stability of the endotracheal tube.

**Comments on teachable moments**

*Teachable moments are not just for nurses new to the critical care setting.* They are also valuable learning opportunities for nurses who have well developed knowledge based on experience with multiple prior cases, yet may need opportunities to refine, challenge, or disconfirm their current beliefs before integrating "new evidence" into their practice. As a point of illustration, it is at the bedside that I have been able to invite experienced nurses to reconsider the practices of routine suctioning based on a timed schedule and the routine instillation of normal saline prior to endotracheal tube suctioning. It is often in the course of caring for patients myself that the experienced nurse will question my practice, thus creating a teachable moment, an opportunity to co-create understanding and reflecting-in-action. I talk aloud about my own clinical reasoning process and model the use of research findings in clinical practice. This strategy has been identified as a strategy to promote evidence-based practice.

In addition, I use teachable moments to help experienced clinicians advance beyond competent practice to proficient or expert practice. Questions such as, "What do you expect from your patient over this shift, tomorrow, and next week?" engages the clinician in projecting patient trajectories and forming conjectures or hypotheses. Asking "What surprised you about this patient, or this situation?" encourages the clinician to consider not only the unique attributes of this patient in relation to what he/she knows about this type of patient, but also other alternative meanings to the event, and possibly even new conclusions. "What did you do differently in this situation?" also encourages the clinician to discover possible cause-effect relationships in her/his actions, while such simple questions as, "What did you see and what did you do in response?" helps to uncover the unnoticed and subtle perceptions that expert clinicians so frequently act upon that contribute to clinical expertise at the bedside.

**Evaluation of the teachable moment**

The teachable moment provides the opportunity for both the teacher and learner to come to an awareness - albeit it potentially different for both individuals - of the breadth and depth of the cues identified as relevant by the clinician and how they were critically appraised in this specific patient situation as to timing and performance of the endotracheal tube suctioning procedure. In just a few minutes, both teacher and learner are able to shed further light on practice expectations for this particular setting and to identify if they were met. Asking the question, "Would you do anything different the next time?" offers the learner the opportunity to reflect on his/her practice and to self identify further learning needs. The door is also open for the teacher to propose further learning strategies, including more teachable moments, as a means to support the clinician in acquiring the knowledge, skill, attitudes, and judgments expected in the specific practice environment.

## References

Benner, P., Hooper-Kyriakidis, P. & Stannard, D. *Clinical wisdom and interventions in critical care: A thinking-in-action approach.* Philadelphia: W.B. Saunders, 1999.

Cranton, P. *Professional development as transformative learning: New perspectives for teachers of adults.* San Francisco, CA: Jossey-Bass, 1996.

Cranton, P. & Carusetta, E. (2004). Perspectives on authenticity in teaching. *Adult Education Quarterly, 55,* 5-22.

Rashotte, J., & Thomas, M. (2001). Teaching clinical judgment: Continuing education for continuous veno-venous hemofiltration (abstract). *DYNAMICS, The Official Journal of the Canadian Association of Critical Care Nurses, 12* (2), 43.

Rashotte, J., & Thomas, M. (2002). Incorporating educational theory into critical care orientation. *The Journal of Continuing Education in Nursing, 33* (3), 131-137.

Schon, D. *Educating the reflective practitioner.* San Francisco, CA: Jossey-Bass, 1987.

Thomas, M. & Fothergill-Bourbonnais, F. (2005). Clinical judgments about endotracheal suctioning: What cues do expert pediatric critical care nurses consider? *Critical Care Nursing Clinics of North America, 17,* 329-340.

Svenson, O. Eliciting and analyzing verbal protocols in process studies of judgment and decision making. In H. Montgomery and O. Svenson, Process and Structure on Human Decision Making, (pp. 65-81). Chichester, UK: John Wiley & Sons, 1989.

Zambok, C. E. & Klein, G. (Eds.) Naturalistic Decision Making, Mahwah, NJ: Lawrence Erlbaum, Publishers. 1997.

# The Clinical Sieve: a Visual Implement to Share the Diagnostic Thinking

## Carlos A. Cuello-García, MD

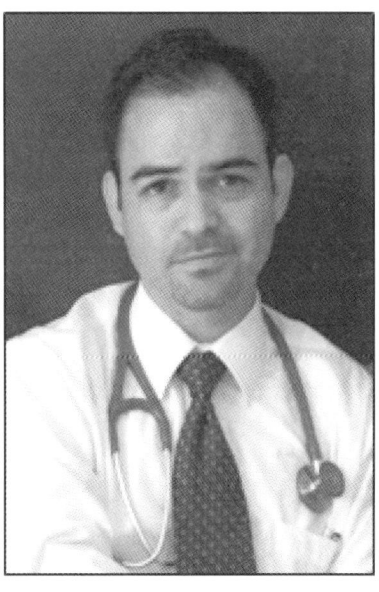

*Dr. Carlos Cuello-García, MD, is a professor of pediatrics and clinical research in the School of Medicine at the Instituto Tecnológico y de Estudios Superiores de Monterrey (ITESM) in Monterrey, Mexico. He directs the Centre for Evidence-Based Medicine (Centro de Medicina Basada en Evidencia del Tecnológico de Monterrey). Dr. Cuello-García uses an interactive pedagogy to teach clinical reasoning using on-line postings of clinical cases. Here he describes a technique for thinking about clinical cases which he terms the "clinical sieve." This session incorporates teaching students about several key diagnostic reasoning concepts: 'sensitivity,' 'specificity,' and 'likelihood ratios.' The exercise is particularly valuable because it uses authentic problem scenarios and can easily adaptable to clinicians in all areas of the health sciences. This type of reasoning context discussed by Dr. Cuello-Garcia (the need for high stakes judgments under conditions of uncertainty) is an example of what has been termed 'naturalistic decision-making.' You can find out more about thinking and decision-making in this type of judgment process in "Naturalistic Decision Making" by Caroline Zsambok and Gary Klein (1997). Thank you, Dr. Cuello-García, for this most interesting clinical session.*

## Background

The clinical sieve was developed in the year 2002 when working with pediatric residents and medical students in morning reports and presentations of clinical cases. In the clinical teaching environment the presentation of clinical cases provides a ready opportunity for the healthcare professional apprentice to deal with the process of decision making. He or she must think about the case and present a list of differential diagnoses based on the data provided from a clinical scenario. Using the list of differential diagnoses, they must then move on to decide which of the entities considered is most likely, and what kind of studies are necessary for reaching a definitive diagnosis. Usually this is time consuming and difficult to present to the tutor or to any other clinician. This decision making process usually involves the use of probabilities of disease or conditions and hence Bayesian reasoning. The clinical sieve can provide a "snapshot" of the thinking process of the clinician at any moment of the "clinician-patient-disease" experience.

## The objectives of the clinical sieve

1. To provide an additional educational tool for the presentation of a clinical case in different settings.

2. To assist health professional apprentices in the resolution and presentation of a clinical case by using probabilities of disease and Bayesian reasoning.

3. To encourage the apprentice to use the most relevant and valid information to decide which diagnostic actions will be taken on a particular case.

4. To facilitate the agreement between clinicians when they face a clinical scenario with several differential diagnoses through the visual evaluation of the most and less likely diagnostic possibilities.

## The student population and settings

Any healthcare professional presenting a case could make use of the clinical sieve. The following examples suggest how it might be used in clinical teaching settings by both clinical professors and health science students and apprentices:

- After morning rounds in a discussion of the differential diagnosis.

- In a short or long case presentation or oral exam with simulated or real patients.

- In problem-based learning teams, when the team is ready to make a visual presentation of the clinical case.

- As part of an interactive lecture as an opportunity to interact with the audience to increase participation in discussion of the differential diagnosis.

All that is needed is a board, a slide show presentation or any visual adjunctive method that nowadays is used as part of the medical educational practice.

## Background to apply the method

The threshold approach by Pauker and Kassirer (1980) is required for the student to understand the process of the clinical sieve. This method is described elsewhere in any evidence-based medicine source (Cuello-Garcia, 2005) and I will give a brief introduction using Figure 1.

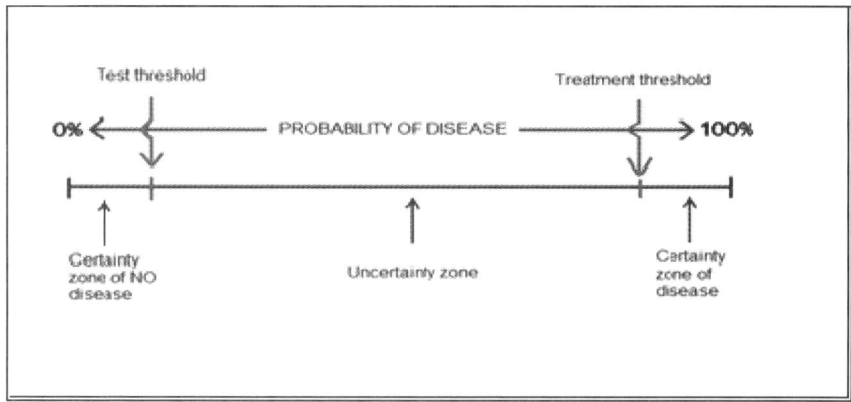

Figure 1: The threshold approach for decision making
(adapted from Pauker and Kassirer, (1980)

In any given clinical case, the probability of a disease or condition must be established by the health professional facing the problem. In Figure 1 you can see a horizontal line depicting the probability of a disease or condition from zero to 100 percent. The line shows that the probabilities are divided into three zones, delimited by two thresholds. Sometimes the probability of a disease is small enough to be in the first zone, this is the *zone of certainty of no-disease* and it means that the probability of disease is low enough that no diagnostic action should be taken at this moment. Certainly the actual probability is not mathematically equal to zero, but rather it is low enough that for the moment it can be treated as zero. Over time and with changing clinical information, the estimates of probability of disease can change, possibly moving the probability from the *zone of certainty of no-disease* to the next zone, *the zone of diagnostic uncertainty* or even to the last zone, *the certainty of disease).*

The movement of the probability of disease from one zone to another occurs as a result of a critical thinking process, interpretation of the available clinical information, analysis of its meaning and the drawing of an inference as to the relevance of the new clinical information to determine which of the differential diagnoses will explain the illness condition. Thus, this decision process involves the critical thinking skills of interpretation, analysis, inference.

For example, consider a patient with mild stomach-ache where the clinician considers the possibility of an appendicitis to be particularly low, and places this probability in the zone of certainty of no-disease so he or she does not have to perform expensive tests at this moment. Now suppose the patient continues with the tummy ache, a mild fever appears and the patient begins vomiting. Interpreting this new clinical information in terms of its relevance for each of the differential diagnoses will lead to a reassessment of the probability of each. By now the clinician may infer that the probability of appendicitis might be greater than before, hence the clinician must consider the performance of a diagnostic action (like a complete blood count, an ultrasound or a computed tomography). The clinician is in doubt (zone of diagnostic uncertainty) whether or not the patient has the clinical entity in question (in this case appendicitis), but considers that the probability of disease is large enough to perform a diagnostic action.

A diagnostic action is any method, procedure, or test performed to diagnose disease, disordered function, or disability; occasionally even time of observation can be considered a diagnostic process. The main objective is to decide which diagnostic tests will be helpful to get the probability of disease to the first zone, where the patient does not have the condition, or on to the certainty of disease zone. In this zone, the patient has enough signs and symptoms supported by laboratory values or other tests that the clinician now can consider the likelihood of a disease as large enough to consider it a certainty and proceed with treatment, preventive care and/or educational plans.

Continuing the example, suppose the patient with the stomach-ache arrives with a classic perforated appendicitis. In this case a clinician would place the patient in the 'certainty of disease zone' immediately, and want to go directly to the operating room and not perform a CT scan or other costly and useless tests. In this case the clinician is relying on the interpretation of the clinical evidence as so highly indicative of the differential diagnosis of appendicitis that he or she feels warranted to infer with confidence that the probability of appendicitis being the true diagnosis can be treated as 100%.

Now consider the two "limits" or thresholds that separate these zones: the first limit is called the test threshold, which is commonly a hazy and clinician-dependent grey zone. It is a decision point and beyond this, a diagnostic action must be taken. A health professional must decide if the disease considered in his or her patient is probable and dangerous enough to perform a diagnostic action, advocating the use of the most relevant and valid information and perhaps group discussion for making this decision. The second is the treatment threshold, also a "grey zone" point of decision for the clinician who must choose to pass this threshold once he or she is ready to initiate treatment on the patient, that is, the probability of the disease is plausible that does not need further tests.

Every diagnostic action has a particular "power" to help clinicians move the probability of the disease forward or backwards; this power is called the likelihood ratio which is obtained from the sensitivity and specificity of the test. The last two values are obtained from clinical studies or textbooks. The formula for calculating the likelihood ratio and interpretation of the various values one obtains as a result of this calculation is described in Table I.

**How to use the clinical sieve in a clinical seminar**

I design the clinical seminar to have two parts: an interactive lecture which I lead, and a subsequent clinical team discussion. I usually use the following clinical vignette when explaining the method, but almost any clinical case can be used in different educational settings. With experience you will be able to decide which topic and with what case scenario the sieve can be used.

> *"Anna is a six- month-old girl that is brought by her parents to the emergency room with fever for the last two days. The past medical history is unremarkable and her immunization schedule is complete. She is attentive, a little fussy but consolable. She doesn't have a toxic appearance but has a temperature of 41°C (rectally), respiratory rate 45 per minute, pulse 120 per minute, oxygen saturation 98% at room air. The rest of her physical examination is unrevealing."*

**Table 1. Formula to obtain the likelihood ratios (LR) for a positive and a negative test and the interpretation based on the results. Sensitivity and specificity must be ≤ 1**

| | |
|---|---|
| **Formula for the Likelihood ratio (LR)** | |
| LR for a positive test result = Sensitivity / 1 − specificity | |
| LR for a negative test result = 1 − sensitivity / specificity | |
| **LR** | **Interpretation** |
| > 10 | Large and often conclusive increase in the likelihood of disease |
| 5 - 10 | Moderate increase in the likelihood of disease |
| 2 - 5 | Small increase in the likelihood of disease |
| 1 - 2 | Minimal increase in the likelihood of disease |
| 1 | **No change in the likelihood of disease** |
| 0.5 - 1.0 | Minimal decrease in the likelihood of disease |
| 0.2 - 0.5 | Small decrease in the likelihood of disease |
| 0.1 - 0.2 | Moderate decrease in the likelihood of disease |
| < 0.1 | Large and often conclusive decrease in the likelihood of disease |

## My interactive clinical lecture

The participants are gathered around a whiteboard and I let them read the case that I prepared (the vignette above). I also ask them to read in advance the topic (in this case, fever in children from 0 to 36 months old) so we could make a more interactive lecture. I start asking them the relevant data from the patient so they can construct a list of problems. This is best performed if they discuss the relevant data, the signs and symptoms and if they can construct a syndrome with the current information. The students review the case and begin to state out loud the problems that they considered to be "activating findings" as described in the work of Custers and co-workers (Custers, Stuyt & De Vries Robbe, 2000) that is, all the information that has diagnostic or therapeutic potential is presented and then portrayed as a problem in a list. Meanwhile I write them down as presented in Figure 2 so the group could see the patient in one piece.

- Chief complaint
  - "fever in my child"

- List of problems
  - Fever >39° C.
  - Irritability.
  - Lack of appetite.

- Syndromes:
  - Fever without localizing signs

**Figure 2: The problem representation**
**The participants obtain a chief complaint, list of problems and syndromes**

After the group completes and evaluate the list of problems, I ask for the differential diagnosis. The apprentices must initiate a brainstorming session. Brainstorming is a technique used to get all potentially relevant ideas on the table. It involves the verbalization of inferences made in response to a particular prompt, in this case the request for possible differential diagnoses. When brainstorming, one does not typically interrupt the process to evaluate or challenge the strength of the inference that led someone to propose an idea, but on occasion this is necessary to avoid the problem of subsequent inferences moving farther and farther away from the objective: to obtain a working list that can guide further thinking.

The tutor could (and usually should) guide the students in a certain order in the process of building the list of problems as in the brainstorming session of the differential diagnoses list. I do this by helping them to organize their thinking into several categories as I write down the conditions as they come up with them. The list of possible diagnoses can be ordered by etiology, organs affected, pathophysiology, anatomy, etc. In this example they preferred to order the list in etiologic groups as they read in a review article last night. I usually end up with a list like the one in Figure 3.

---

**List of Possible Diagnoses**

- Serious bacterial infections.
    - Occult pneumococcal bacteremia.
    - Urinary tract infection.
    - Pneumonia.
    - Gastroenteritis
    - CNS infections
- Viral infections.
    - Enterovirus
    - Respiratory syncytial virus
    - Parainfluenza
    - Dengue
    - Measles
    - SARS
- Others
    - Kawasaki syndrome

---

FIGURE 3: DIFFERENTIAL DIAGNOSES LIST

In the next step I say "Determine the probability of every condition that you considered in your patient (in this case, Anna)". I encourage the team to ask: "What is the probability of occult bacteremia?" "What about the probability of a urinary tract infection? Meningitis? Pneumonia?" "Briefly describe each one of the diseases" "Which is more likely?" "Which is more dangerous?" "How would you manage the thresholds for each one of them? Think and apply the test threshold in each possibility." "Is it possible that the patient could have two or more clinical entities explaining the process?" In each case I require them to explain their answers.

Each of these questions initiates a thinking and decision process that demands the use of critical thinking skills, in this case emphasizing the skills of *analysis, inference* and *explanation*. The assignment of probability is another critical thinking process, emphasizing the skills of *analysis, inference* and *evaluation*.

**Clinical Team Discussion:**
At this point the visual part and the discussion begins. The group has to get to an agreement by applying the threshold method that we described earlier to each of the diagnostic possibilities.

Which entities are probable and dangerous enough to pass to the uncertainty zone (*analysis* and *inference*)? This question is usually a clinical challenge and it's a very important step in the whole process. Keep in mind that the team will have to perform a diagnostic action if the probability of disease is in the uncertainty zone. By diagnostic action I mean anything from a dangerous, costly and uncomfortable procedure (like a lumbar puncture or a cardiac catheterisation) to a simple and inexpensive process (like just leaving the patient in the observation room). This question makes the student consider patient preferences and values, solid clinical evidence and their own clinical experience by balancing costs, pain and time using the critical thinking skills of *evaluation* and *explanation*. The team will ponder their own efficacy, efficiency and effectiveness.

Using defining and discriminating features the team begins to discuss why this patient could have or not have each one of the diseases that they considered in their differential diagnosis, and how likely is each one of them. As they tell me I write a line in front of every condition and they advise me how long (probable) or short must be, and if the possibility is large enough to "pass" to the uncertainty zone or even to the certainty zone of disease. In the course of this discussion they must say what evidence they are using to determine the length of the line (answering the key critical thinking questions: "Why do I/you come to this conclusion"). According to the probabilities that they considered after activating their previous knowledge based on a recent review, they finally decided that Figure 4 would be the initial visualization of the problem.

As you can note, according to the students appreciation, there are several diagnostic possibilities that they have placed in the uncertainty zone, and hence they will ask for a diagnostic action only for those probabilities that are positioned in this area. At this moment, the team sees a patient with a viral infection as the most likely explanation for her problems, but they cannot reject the possibility of a urinary tract infection or an occult bacteremia, because they presented evidence that there is a 7% and 3% chance of them respectively. For them this probability was high enough to pass these two conditions to the uncertainty zone, but it was not the case for the other conditions, at least not for the moment (for example, they did not consider to perform a lumbar puncture to rule out meningitis or a chest x-ray for pneumonia). The next step is to perform

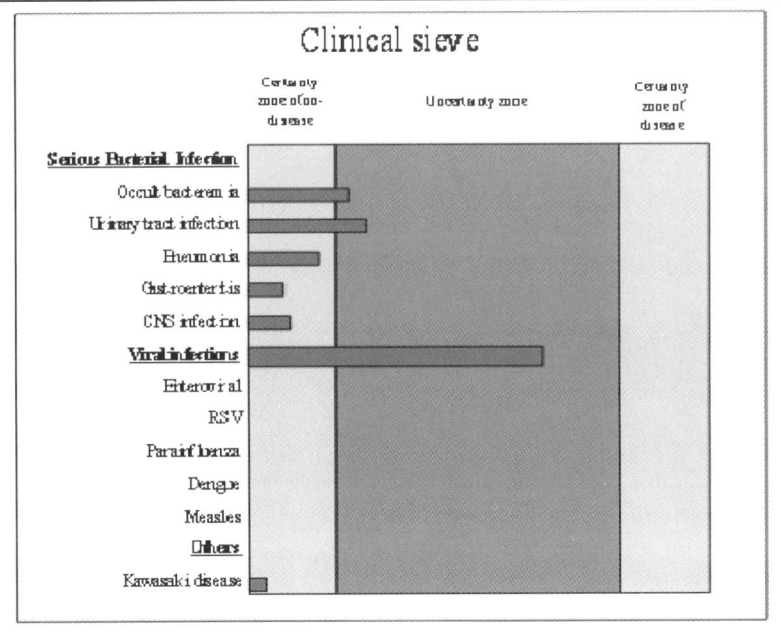

**Figure 4: Clinical sieve, first agreement by the students.**

**Important note:** for visual reasons, the lines of the test and treatment threshold are represented as two vertical lines, but these thresholds are different in every diagnostic possibility (*i.e.*, the occult bacteremia threshold might be low because it is a precarious entity, contrary to the viral infection which is harmless, so its threshold could be more relaxed)

the diagnostic actions for the conditions in the uncertainty zone, but as in the previous step, they have to consider availability of the test, costs, pain, timing, diagnostic accuracy and easiness for the patient or family.

When defining the diagnostic actions for each condition in the uncertainty zone, they decided that a complete blood count, a blood culture, urinalysis and a urine culture would be sufficient for the moment. Some times one student might ask for a completely out of context test (for example, a Widal test for ruling out a typhoid fever) but he or she would be questioned by the rest of the group when they do not see this disease as part of the sieve and even if it was, they would not put it into the uncertainty zone. The group process offers the opportunity for the demand for a critical thinking explanation of this conclusion to come from the learner rather than the professor. The group makes the point that if, at this point, the speaker would like a new diagnosis (and therefore a new test) in the uncertainty zone, they will have to give solid data to back their opinion.

Sometimes, evidence about a condition or hypothesis will be limited, and clinical intuition could be used at this point in the clinical sieve and give the team a moment to reconsider the case and critically think about the possibility of any bias or heuristic that any clinician in a real life case would use. Experienced clinicians often unconsciously use several, combined analytic and non-analytic strategies to solve clinical problems suggesting a high degree of mental flexibility and adaptability in clinical reasoning (Bowen, 2006), and the expert could discuss along with the team how she or he would have portrayed the differential diagnosis in the sieve and why. When the evidence (i.e., diagnostic accuracy, sensitivity or specificity) about a given diagnostic test is not available at all, the team should not seen this as a burden but as an opportunity to continue the search for the truth and promote their interest for clinical research.

**Figure 5: Diagnostic actions taken by the students and test results with their respective likelihood ratios (LR).**

CBC= complete blood count. WBC, white blood cells. ANC, absolute neutrophil count. N.A., not available. L.E., leukocyte esterase.

| Diagnostic actions | | | |
|---|---|---|---|
| Test | Results | LR Positive Test | LR Negative Test |
| CBC | WBC 18,000 | 3.7 | N.A. |
| | ANC 12,000 | 3.5 | N.A. |
| Urinalysis | Gram stain is positive | 18 | N.A. |
| | 15 wbc/mm$^3$ | 7 | N.A. |
| | LE and nitrites negative | N.A. | 0.5 |
| Blood culture | N.A. | N.A. | N.A. |
| Urine culture (bladder catheterization) | N.A. | N.A. | N.A. |

During the team discussion, I have been generating the list of the clinical tests that will be requested by the team as a result of the assigned probabilities of each differential diagnosis in the uncertainty zone. My job is also to guide the discussion when necessary be sure that the final list approximates the optimal list of the experienced clinician. When possible, the team (or the tutor) provides the value of the likelihood ratio obtained from the sensitivity and specificity from clinical trials or from textbooks. This encourages the team to ask good clinical questions and scarch for the most valid and relevant information. The timing of this clinical team discussion, searching to answer the clinical questions in this case, is the decision of the tutor. On occasion, I split the lecture into two parts to give the student time to search for the data between class sessions. Once the request for diagnostic tests is complete, I expose the results for the case (Figure 5).

In the next step the team must develop a second sieve depicting how their diagnostic possibilities changed based on the present evidence. At this point, altogether they will apply Bayesian reasoning, that is, using the present evidence (the likelihood ratios of the tests) to move the pre-test probabilities after a diagnostic test result is presented. For example, in the case of a urinary tract infection, the urinalysis test shows a positive gram stain. One of the students had read (and showed an article) that a positive gram stain has a likelihood ratio of 18. This evidence is strong enough to move forward the probability of a urinary tract infection (see Table I). If the tutor or the team would like to be more specific they could use the nomogram of Fagan to accomplish an exact result of the post-test probability (Fagan, 1975).

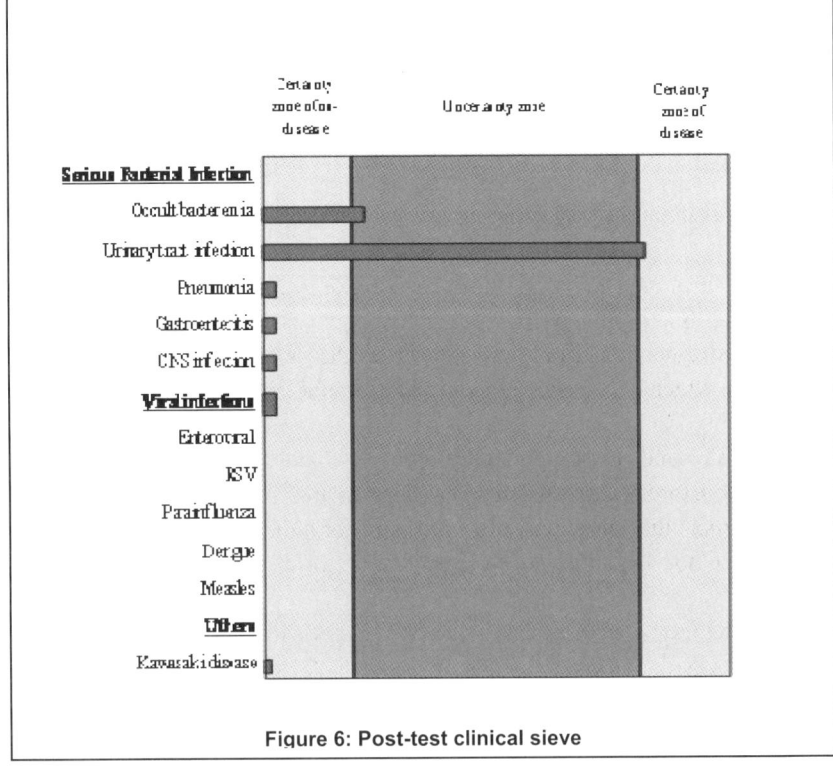

Figure 6: Post-test clinical sieve

The tutor should now ask the team: "How have these test results changed your view?" "What do you think now?" "How are you thinking at this moment about this patient?" "Which diagnoses will you move forward and how will you move them?" "Do we need more tests or are we ready to move on to determining the treatment?" "Show me how you would sketch the clinical sieve now"

The team usually ends up with a schematic like the one in Figure 6, and as expected, the probability of a urinary tract infection (UTI) is in the certainty zone of disease, that is, the team is sufficiently sure about this diagnosis that is ready to move to the treatment plans, thanks to the high likelihood ratio given by the positive gram stain. The LR positive of 18 gave a post-test probability of 60% for the patient of having a UTI.

Viewing the second sieve the team is not yet sure if the patient has bacteremia, thus they will have to wait for the results of the blood culture. Concerning the UTI, they will not wait for the results of the urine culture just as they considered a 60% chance of the disease is enough to initiate the antibiotic (i.e., prophylaxis). The lecture can continue from here, discussing the other part of the therapeutic plans, which include preventive, educational and further diagnostic plans.

**Conclusion**

In real life a clinician almost never will have a 100% assurance about a diagnosis, but certainly he or she will almost be sure about one or two possibilities in a given case. Clinicians mostly use some heuristic to rapidly explain a clinical problem. Resolving a clinical case is a complex process involving a high level of meta-cognitive events.

Any health professional in the teaching environment could make use of the clinical sieve as a visual tool for sharing the diagnostic process. It blends clinical reality and diagnostic reasoning, encouraging the use of clinical judgment and evidence on which diagnostic tests would be helpful, and attaining agreement by scientific discussion among health-care professionals. In terms of critical thinking, it demands reason-giving by the thinker and the thinking team at each stage of the exercise. It can help clinicians in training to interpret evidence, graphics, probability questions, pros and cons for a diagnostic test and drawing judicious and non-fallacious conclusions.

Learners should be encouraged to read about their patients' problems and present the situation to their teachers in a way that promote the skills of critical thinking, rather than to present clinical cases without context and read about topics in a rote-memorization fashion.

## References

Bowen, J. L. (2006). Educational strategies to promote clinical diagnostic reasoning. *New England Journal of Medicine,* 355, 2217-2225.

Cuello-Garcia, C. (2005). Sharing the diagnostic process in the clinical teaching environment: a case study. *Journal of Continuing Education in the Health Professions,* 25(4), 231-239.

Custers, E.J., Stuyt, P.M., De Vries, & Robbe, P. F. (2000). Clinical problem analysis (CPA): a systematic approach to teaching complex medical problem solving. *Academic Medicine,* 75(3), 291-297.

Fagan, T. J. (1975). Letter: Nomogram for Bayes theorem. *New England Journal of Medicine,* 293, 257.

Pauker, S.G. & Kassirer, J. P. (1980). The threshold approach to clinical decision making. *New England Journal of Medicine,* 302, 1109-1117.

# Using Short Cases to Teach Thinking

## *Marilyn H. Oermann*

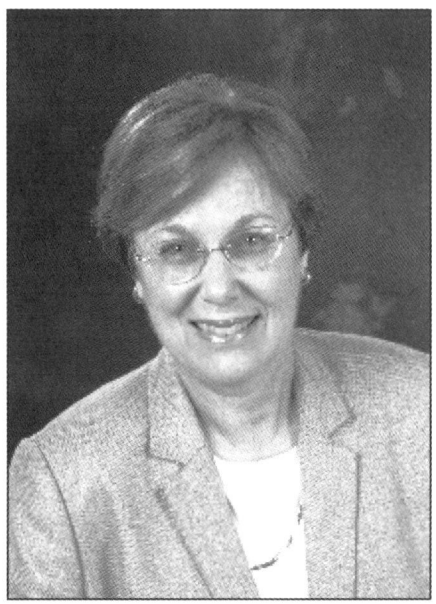

*Dr. Marilyn Oermann is Professor and Academic Division Chair at the University of North Carolina at Chapel Hill, a Fellow in the American Academy of Nursing, and the editor of the 2008 "Annual Review of Nursing Education," published by Springer Publishing Company. She has authored a collection of theoretical papers that constitutes one of Nursing's best collections on theory based teaching and learning, and curriculum assessment. Her award winning book entitled "Evaluation and Testing in Nursing Education" and several others most relevant for critical thinking and clinical judgment are listed at the end of this chapter.*

*In the following chapter Dr. Oermann shares her expertise on the use of short clinical cases to externalize and evaluate evidence of critical thinking in her nursing students. Her discussion of the need to think aloud for students is exactly true, and the practice of doing so is one of the most valuable gift that can be offered to the clinical student by an expert critical thinker and diagnostician. The "think aloud" method was first described in 1920 by behaviorist John Watson as the way to learn more about how people think. We believe that cultivating this habit of mind is also one of the most helpful strategies for growing one's critical thinking skills at any age.*

### Class Session and Students:

This example demonstrates the use of short cases, integrated in a nursing class, for promoting the development of critical thinking skills. Short cases, which apply concepts being learned to hypothetical clinical situations, provide an opportunity for students to identify varied patient problems, propose multiple alternatives for resolving them, decide on the best approach from among those alternatives, and develop a rationale to support their thinking. Short cases can be developed for any nursing class, in pre-licensure through graduate programs, and this teaching method is easily adapted for classes in other health sciences.

**The Goal of the Class Session:**

My goal for this type of class session is to provide experiences for students to carry out in depth analysis of clinical cases. An in depth analysis would include: identifying possible problems that a patient might experience, exploring multiple alternatives for resolving them, comparing alternatives, and making decisions about the best approaches in consideration of i what is known about the case. All of these cognitive exercises involve critical thinking and can be accomplished through the use of the 'short case.' A short case is a simulated clinical situation, but one with all the characteristics of an authentic clinical case. The short case also assists students to practice applying content learned in class and through readings to simulated clinical situations, and later to actual clinical cases. This class guides students in the practice of their critical thinking skills with an emphasis on interpretation, analysis, and inference skills. These skills can be seen in the learning objectives below.

**Learning Objectives:**

Students who participate in this class will be able to:
- Identify multiple patient problems using concepts learned in class.
  (Emphasis: interpretation and analysis).
- Propose alternative approaches that might be used to resolve those problems.
  (Emphasis: inference and explanation).
- Arrive at an informed decision about the best approaches to use in the simulated case situation.
  (Emphasis: inference, and evaluation).
- Develop a rationale that supports their thinking and decisions
  (Emphasis: analysis and explanation).

**What I do Before Class Begins:** As I prepare my notes for class, I identify the critical thinking skills to be developed and if the case will focus on (a) identifying multiple patient problems using concepts learned in class or (b) proposing alternate approaches that might be used in the clinical scenario. I then write short cases with open ended questions for the class. For each class session, I always bring additional short cases for use if students have difficulty applying new concepts to the scenarios and for small group work if our discussion ends early. For this session, I developed four cases on the care of patients with chronic pulmonary problems.

## My example cases for this lesson:
### Table 1. Sample Short Cases for Teaching Skills of Interpretation, Analysis, and Inference

| CASE | QUESTIONS |
|------|-----------|
| Your elderly patient with severe COPD is developing sores on his back but refuses to get out of bed. He asks you to please leave him sleep. | 1. What is the priority problem in this case that needs to be solved? Why do you think this is the priority?<br><br>2. What additional data would you collect before you planned your nursing care? Why is this information critical to your decision making? |
| Your patient in the clinic has an elevated temperature, a sore throat, and a cough. | 1. What additional information would you collect *first* and why?<br><br>2. Name 2 possible problems that could occur with these symptoms. For each problem identify lab values that you would expect. Which of these problems seems most likely and why?<br><br>3. A few days later the patient returns to the clinic. Propose a new symptom that would alter your decision about the problem you listed in #2. |
| Mrs. J, your 70-year-old patient with pneumonia, appears to be coughing more than the nurse indicated in the change-of-shift report. You check the medical record, and the nurse who cared for Mrs. J for the last 2 days noted that the patient was "coughing more" and was "too short of breath to get out of bed." As a result the nurse kept Mrs. J in bed for that time period. | 1. Do you agree with this plan of care? Why or why not?<br><br>2. What information would you look for the medical record? Record what you found and develop a new plan of care. Provide a rationale including evidence for your approaches. |
| You are discharging a 7-year-old child who had been admitted following an asthma attack. In talking with the mother, you learn that the child has been seen in the Emergency Department at your hospital and elsewhere nearly monthly for the last year. | 1. What are 2 different actions you could take at this time?<br><br>2. Which of these would you do and why? |

## How I write the cases
Each case usually has two parts: a brief description of a patient situation that relates to the concepts presented in the class, and open-ended questions about the case for students to answer in small groups. I keep the case descriptions short to avoid directing student thinking in advance toward a particular problem or approach. Since this is a teaching strategy used throughout the course, the cases increase in complexity over a period of time and the focus (identifying potential problems or alternatives) varies. In developing these cases, I also integrate concepts learned in prior courses.

The questions that are developed for the case depend on the outcomes of thinking (e.g., interpretation, analysis, and inference) that the teacher is intending to promote. For example, questions can ask students to identify all possible problems from the data presented in the case and how a clinician would decide which problem is the priority problem. Or they might ask students to propose multiple alternatives for resolving a problem and then to determine the best approach to use. For all answers, students provide a rationale for their thinking.

## How I teach this lesson
To prepare students for how short cases are used in the course, I begin one of the first class sessions with a sample case that presents problems and approaches that they have learned in a prior nursing course. I analyze the case for students, "thinking aloud" about potential problems in the case scenario, significant cues, alternate approaches to consider, what I would decide for this patient, and why. In this way I can model thinking step-by-step through the case.

After presenting theoretical information about a patient condition, I use the short cases that apply this new information to a simulated client situation. Students receive different cases to analyze, all of which relate to the clinical condition presented in that class and foster development of critical thinking. Students divide into small groups, with three or four students in each group, or when I am teaching larger classes in classrooms with immovable seats, they work in pairs with the student sitting next to them. I only give them a limited amount of time (e.g., 5 minutes) to read the case and answer the questions. I limit the time so students keep their discussion focused on the case and the intended outcomes of their group work. A short time frame also simulates actual clinical practice where health professionals need to identify quickly the critical features of a patient situation (i.e., a case) and decide what to do. Students must come to a group consensus about their answers to questions related to the case.

In small classes, one student from the group presents the case and answers to the entire class. The other students then critique the responses and suggest other possibilities. In large classes, I randomly choose students to report their answers to the group. With all cases, students must explain how they arrived at their decisions and their reasoning.

**What I Expect from the Class Participants**
In small group classrooms, I expect each student to make a contribution to the analysis of and discussion about the case. Although one student may emerge as a leader, this exercise is a group activity requiring cooperation and collaboration. When the cases focus on problem identification, I expect students to think about the data in the case, propose varied problems that might be possible, and explain how they would decide on the problem. In their discussions students should identify significant cues in the case that influenced their thinking and explain why the cues are significant.

If the questions for the case ask about interventions, I expect students to generate multiple approaches that could be used. Using what they know and what they are learning in class, I want them to weigh the benefits and costs of each potential approach, and decide as a group which approaches would be "best." Students must come to group consensus, which encourages students to explain and support their thinking to the group.

**The Student Work Product**
Assessment of student critical thinking skills as applied to clinical practice occurs in two forms: through classroom testing using higher level items and clinical evaluation. Higher level test items present new information for interpretation and analysis by students; with these items, students cannot memorize an answer but need to analyze the case and the new data in it. While difficult, these higher level items assess students' skill in interpretation, analysis, and inference. Figure 1 shows two examples of test items for evaluating the learning outcomes of this class session follow. The first one is an essay item and the second example uses a modification of the multiple-choice format.

> **Question 1:** You are a registered nurse providing consultation through a nurse telephone service for a group of pediatricians. You receive a call from a mother about her daughter's "breathing problems" and "stomach cramps." The mother tells you that her daughter has asthma and allergies.
>
> 1. What questions would you ask the mother? Why are these questions critical to your decision making?
> 2. Add new data to this case based on the mother's answers to your questions. What are potential problems of the daughter? Describe how you arrived at these conclusions.
>
> **Question 2:** This is another busy day in the Emergency Department where you work as a registered nurse. You receive report on the following 4 patients for whom you are responsible. Which of these patients would you observe first?
>
> 1. An 82-year-old with respiratory symptoms including cough, shortness of breath, and wheezing.
> 2. A 70-year-old with COPD who is apparently confused.
> 3. A 20-year-old with a pneumothorax and chest tubes following a motorcycle accident.
> 4. A 6-year-old following an asthma attack.
>
> Provide an explanation of your reasons for choosing that patient to observe first.

**Figure 1:**

**Test items that can be used to assess learning in this class session**

The most important assessment, though, is in the practice setting. In clinical practice students can be observed on their competency in interpreting patient data, examining evidence, identifying possible problems, suggesting alternate approaches that might be effective for their patients, and evaluating those approaches to decide on the best possible ones.

### Feedback from Students

Student feedback about the short cases is consistently positive. Not only do students recognize the importance of learning how to apply concepts from class to patient situations, in preparing them for future practice, they comment frequently on the value of group discussion of these cases. By analyzing cases in small groups, students learn from one another and have a safe environment to discuss their thinking and reasoning. Additionally, analyzing short cases in small groups provides for active learning in class, which maintains student interest.

## References:

Gaberson, K., & Oermann, M.H.. Case Method, Case Study, and Grand Rounds. In *Clinical teaching strategies in nursing* (2nd Ed.). New York: Springer, 2007.

Oermann, M.H. (1997). Evaluating critical thinking in clinical practice. *Nurse Educator, 22*(5), 25-28.

Oermann, M.H. (1998). How to assess critical thinking in clinical practice. *Dimensions of Critical Care Nursing*, 17, 322-327.

Oermann, M. H. (2004). Using active learning in lecture: Best of "both worlds." *Journal of Nursing Education Scholarship, 1*(1), 1-11.
    Available at http://www.bepress.com/ijnes/vol1/iss1/art1

Oermann, M.H. (2006). Short written assignments for clinical nursing courses. *Nurse Educator*, *31*(5), 228-231.

Oermann, M.H., & Gaberson, K. Evaluation of Higher-Level Learning, Problem Solving, and Critical Thinking. In, *Evaluation and testing in nursing education,* (2nd Ed.). New York: Springer, 2006.

Oermann, M.H., Truesdell, S., & Ziolkowski, L. (2000). Strategy to assess, develop, and evaluate critical thinking. *Journal of Continuing Education in Nursing,* 31, 155-160.

# Case Study Tutorial with Guided Reasoning: Developing Self Evaluation of Critical Thinking and Clinical Reasoning Skills

## Wolter Paans, Rose M.B. Nieweg, Marleen Vermeulen, & Frans van der Werf

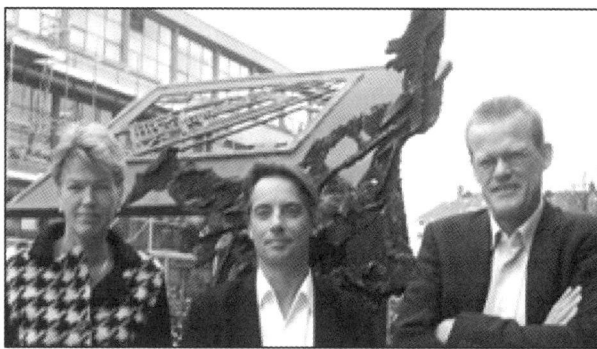

*These authors are members of the collaborative group "Critical Thinking in Nursing in the Netherlands," at the Hanze University in Groningen and at Kairos (Rotterdam) in the Netherlands.*

Hanze University Groningen is one of the largest and comprehensive universities of professional education and applied sciences in the Netherlands. Internationalization is a particular goal of the School of Nursing at Hanze University. Every year the Academy of Nursing organizes an "International Intensive Programme." Dutch students and tutors from Hanze work together with colleagues and students from Finland, Sweden, Norway, the Czech Republic, Latvia, Lithuania, Spain, Scotland and United States. Kairos is a consultancy company, specialized in innovation, training and organizational development in health care in the Netherlands.

Professor Walter Paans collaborated on the Dutch translation of the Health Sciences Reasoning Test (HSRT) used widely to assess critical thinking skills in health science students and practitioners. Here, he and his colleagues use case studies to train their students in the skills of analysis and metacogntive reflection.

## Introduction

We title this lesson: "Critical thinking and clinical reasoning: the Case of Mrs. A." It is intended for first or second year nursing students in a Bachelor degree program here at Hanze University but we think it would be well received by health science students anywhere. We teach this case study exercise in a small seminar class of twelve students. In order for students to benefit maximally from the case, we ask them to read ahead and to prepare themselves for this session by acquiring basic knowledge in three areas: logical reasoning (deductive and inductive reasoning, deductive abduction, and the common fallacies); the nursing process and reporting of diagnoses; and diabetes mellitus, type 1.

## The learning objectives

Students completing this session will be able to:
- Analyze and interpret the clinical case
- Write accurate diagnoses
- Explain the thinking process underpinning the diagnoses being made
- Critically reflect on their personal diagnostic reasoning, analyzing and evaluating the quality of their reasoning skills
- Identify areas of personal development to improve diagnostic reasoning

## How we teach this lesson

The case study supposes that a nurse conducts a patient assessment interview using Gordon's framework (Gordon, 1994). Gordon's Functional Health Patterns Framework has eleven subject areas directing the collect of patient data about common patterns of behaviour that contribute to health, quality of life and the achievement of human potential. The framework is similar to others used in patient intake interviews to guide the clinician to conduct a comprehensive assessment. We prepare copies in advance for each of the students of what appears to be a completed and transcribed interview. In this case example, the interview has been conducted with a client named 'Mrs. A.' who has diabetes mellitus, type 1. Gordon's eleven patterns can be found as the lay-out of a script of the interview. The interview is displayed over the next few pages as Figure 1: "Interview with Mrs. A."

**Figure 1 "Interview with Mrs. A"**

**1. Health perception/health management**
*Can you tell me how you are doing?*
- Reasonably well under the circumstances.

*Reasonably well under the circumstances?*
- Yes, I want to go home as soon as I can. There is plenty of work for me to do, and there's no one to help me do it.

*Do you know why you were admitted?*
- Yes, apparently I fell asleep and the people at the workshop weren't able to wake me. They know I am a diabetic, so they are quick to think it's got something to do with that.

*Can you tell me what I can do for you?*

- Yes, you can ask if my new glasses have already arrived. I've got poor eyesight, you know. It's gone worse in recent years.

*Is there anything else I can do for you?*
- No, I don't think so. I'll give the garage a call later on, to make sure that they take care of things.

*Do you ever feel down or depressed?*
- No, not really. Well, I'm on my own, you know. I live on the premises of the *garage; there are plenty of people I can talk to. But at night, you're on your own again, aren't you. And after a marriage of twenty years, that's not always easy. And then there's the divorce. Most contacts are about work only.*

*Are you in touch with your GP or with a diabetes nurse?*
- No, I take care of everything myself; I can cope. Although sometimes I'm a bit careless.

*What about your therapy management (compliance)?*
- Determining my blood sugar level, injecting the insulin, I do it myself; admittedly not always at the correct time. And I take blood samples, which isn't something I enjoy. Sometimes I inject insulin without first determining the blood sugar level. I just inject the same amount as the days before.

*Does that go well?*
- More or less the same; I am less accurate because I don't consider it all that important. It's always the same anyway. If it doesn't go well, I eat a bit more or inject a bit more insulin. I go by my feeling.

## 2. Nutritional/metabolic

*How about eating and drinking?*
- I eat and drink healthy, not too much, and not too little; I stick to my diet. The wife of one of my employees cooks for me; I pay her for it. And I eat at the garage canteen. Not always in time, I admit. I regulate it with the insulin. I don't lose weight and I don't put on weight. I just don't take the time to eat. And when I do eat, I'm usually on my own ...

*Do you drink alcohol?*
- No, actually I never drink. Except for yesterday. I was sitting at the desk and I found a bottle of blackcurrant gin. I used to drink it at the end of the afternoon. Just one glass before dinner. Yesterday I thought: "I'll have a couple". So, I fell asleep... I'm not into drugs or anything like that. I don't smoke either.

## 3. Elimination

*Do you have any problems with the bowels? Do you have to pass water often?*
- No problems; nothing special.

## 4. Activity/exercise pattern

*How about your physical appearance?*
- I do everything myself; I don't need any help. Sometimes when I feel listless and tired it takes me more time to take care of things. I have the laundry done every two weeks. I don't mind the odd spot or other. Nobody's bothered anyway. Actually, I don't always see it.

*Do you perspire a lot?*
-No, I don't think so.

*Do you practise a sport? How about regular physical exercise?*
- I always enjoyed diving in the Dutch Antilles. I don't do it anymore. I can hardly see under water. I like to read. I can read reasonably well with extra reading glasses. I get plenty of exercise at work.

### 5. Sleep/rest
*Do you enjoy a good night's sleep?*
- I sleep enough. Go to bed in time. I make sure that I have finished work at 7. Sometimes I feel tired and listless in between. It annoys me. I'm also annoyed by small things. I'll be yawning by the end of the afternoon.

*How long have you been bothered by tiredness?*
- Since a couple of weeks

### 6. Cognitive/perceptual
*What can you say about your eyesight?*
- Yes, can you ask if my new glasses have arrived? I don't see well, you know. It's grown worse in recent years. I'm worried about my eyesight; I'm afraid that it'll get worse and I won't be able to see. And it also scared me that they couldn't wake me. Suppose they hadn't found me … On the other hand, who cares?

*Do you have any small wounds, infections? And if yes, do they hurt?*
- A year ago, I had a superficial burn after an accident at work. It took a long time to heal. The skin was also inflamed for a while. It's better now. I just didn't realise my left foot was so close to that gas flame. An employee quickly pulled me away. I have a few small wounds on my feet, they heal slowly; they feel a bit awkward.

### 7. Self-perception/self-concept
*How did things used to be as far as your illness was concerned? / What about your medical history?*
- I've known about my diabetes since I was twelve. It sometimes bothered me when I couldn't control it. Things were different in those days. Many visits to the GP, a long time in the waiting room and still not feeling well. And you weren't allowed to eat the things you liked. Generally speaking, I can handle it better now, although lately I tend to neglect it sometimes. Although I'm aware of that. I'm never really ill and there's nothing that makes me visit the doctor.

*How do you cope with your illness?*
- I more or less take care of everything myself. No problem. Perhaps sometimes I'm a bit careless.

*Are you properly informed about diabetes?*
- I believe I am; after all these years, you think you should know about it. You know what you are supposed to do, but you don't always do it.

### 8. Roles/relationship
*Can they get along without you at work?*
- Sure, for a short time; I have good employees; things at the garage will run their course. It's a family business. Until recently, I used to run things with my husband. But now I am on my own. Sometimes things get busy, because many financial things need to be done. And I like to lend a hand with the sorting work.

*You are on your own?*

- Yes, I'm in a divorce procedure. My husband couldn't stand working in the garage any longer and liked to live in the city... It's a bit of a long-drawn procedure; but I'd prefer not to say much about it. But, well, alone is still alone, and sometimes I think: 'why am I doing it?'

*Do you have any social contacts?*
- Plenty, every day; staff and customers. My son is in Aruba, I only see him about three times a year. Pity. I really miss him, especially at times like these. Apart from that, nobody actually. My staff see me as a good boss, I think, although sometimes I can be rather curt and irritated. More so than in the past, though. It's not easy to get to know new people when you have to run your own business.

*Do you worry about the business?*
- No, economically things are reasonably stable. We have to work hard. Everyone is pulling their weight.

### 9. Sexuality/reproductive
*Are there any problems, sexually?*
- I miss my husband, from a relational point of view; sexually it's less important. It was more important to my husband. Our marriage had lost much of its excitement in that area; I didn't really mind.

### 10. Coping/stress tolerance
*Do you feel any stress?*
- No, I don't feel any stress. Sometimes it's very busy at work but that's a pleasant activity. I can easily handle the work. At least, if I have the energy.

### 11. Value/belief
*Do you have a special belief or religious conviction we should take account of?*
- No, I don't.

*End of interview*

---

In this small seminar session, we begin the lesson by explaining that this is a four part exercise that will be completed over several hours. The lesson involves the analysis of a case history that will be partly dealt with individually and partly in pairs. To help the lesson unfold we have divided the clinical reasoning activities into five sections, and we prepare in advance some instructions to guide the students to work thoughtfully through each to complete the lesson. These instructions are shown sequentially in Figures 2 through 5. While some of the instructions can be delivered orally, we've included them in written form here. Some of the reasoning exercises are done individually, some in small groups and some in the full seminar group.

**Preconditions**

For this assignment you will need a study room for a period of three hours and a (student) colleague with whom you get along well. The room should have at least one large table or two small tables and two chairs. Have pen and paper at the ready. You will also be highly inclined to test your diagnostic reasoning in order to improve your nursing care skills.

You should have a case, an assignments guide and an anamnesis interview conducted using Gordon's framework. The interview provides the case data you will need for the assignments.

**Method**

First read assignments 1 to 5, the case and the script before you start to answer the questions asked in the assignments. Assignment 1 (1a to 1e) is carried out individually, without consulting your colleague (45 minutes). The remaining assignments (2 to 5) are carried with your colleague (45 minutes).This is followed by the plenary discussion afterwards (60 minutes).

For the purpose of this assignment, imagine the following: your colleague has conducted an anamnesis interview with a patient. However, just before your colleague is about to write down the diagnoses, he is called away to resuscitate another patient. You come to see the patient and discover your colleague's notes. Use the notes that your colleague has written down (in this instance the case with the script) to analyze the case. Since you do not want the patient to have to discuss his case history all over again, confine yourself to the information you have.

The aim of the assignment is for you to use the knowledge you have to analyze the case with a colleague and determine the appropriate diagnoses. You will also analyze what your own diagnostic reasoning skills are and identify areas of personal development that may help you improve your diagnostic skills in your own clinical practice. The starting point is to combine logical reasoning with background information on how to make diagnoses.

Figure 2: Instructions for this case study lesson

As we typically have 12 students in the group, we will have six pairs of students. This case study exercise asks students to consider information gathered in an assessment interview. We also explain that there will be time afterwards for the case to be discussed with the teacher and with the full group. During this discussion, the teacher will put critical questions to the students. The teacher will, as it were, act as a catalyst to facilitate the discussion in a Socratic dialogue with the students. The idea is that in the discussion the diagnoses that are being made are substantiated through the students' responses to this questioning.

## Background

Profile: woman; age: 60 years. Admitted to hospital yesterday afternoon, internal medicine ward. At the moment, just after breakfast, out of bed, waiting for an interview with the nurse.

Profession: director-owner of a garage in the region. Works long hours. Tries to take one day a week off but this is not always possible due to pressure of work and demanding customers. Sometimes also lends a hand in the workshop for light sorting work.

Home situation: is in the middle of a divorce procedure, which has been dragging on for a long time. Lives alone in an apartment on the garage premises.

Children: 1 grown-up son, no grandchildren. The son lives on Aruba, the Netherlands Antilles.

Hobbies: reading regional novels or romantic books, diving.

## History

Diabetes patient (type 1) since the age of 12. It took years for the blood sugar level to stabilise and the proper medication to be prescribed. From her fiftieth, the blood sugar level has been stable. The patient herself believes that she can live with diabetes. She wears glasses. Without glasses she sees only outlines.

Two months ago, in the workshop, she suffered slight burns on her left foot without feeling anything. Fortunately, an employee intervened in time.

## Current situation

Yesterday Mrs. A. was urgently admitted to hospital after an employee had found her sleeping. He was unable to wake her. The ambulance staff found that she was unconscious and smelled of alcohol.

Today she is calm and clear.

## Additional information

Patient's appearance: patient's clothes are normally tidy but now she looks untidy: buttons are missing, spots on shawl, shoelaces are undone.

Medication used: Insulin (administered with insulin pin twice a day). She controls the dose herself on the basis of the blood sugar level. She admits that she has been rather careless with this recently; yesterday afternoon she did not inject any insulin because she had fallen asleep after drinking three glasses of blackcurrant gin in a short time (something she normally never does).

Appointments with GP: blood sugar checks somewhat neglected recently.

**Figure 3: The Case of Mrs. A, a patient known to have diabetes**

**Work individually to respond to the following questions:**

**Making diagnoses**

1. Using the case and the script, analyze the diagnoses relevant to nursing and write them down as accurately as possible.

    1a- Underpin each diagnosis you have made with argumentation; Write down in just a few words why you believe it to be a diagnosis.

    1b- Classify each diagnosis as a 'potential diagnoses' or an 'actual diagnoses.'

    1c- For each actual diagnosis, indicate how certain you are about the diagnosis made, using the following symbols:
        ++     very certain
        +      certain
        +/ -   reasonably certain
        –      uncertain
        - -    very uncertain
    Critically reason your choice.

    1d- If the case and the script offer insufficient information for you to be certain to very certain about each of these actual diagnoses, what would you do to become more certain about the diagnosis. Write down the answer in a few words.

    1e- On the basis of the script, give a value judgement about the quality of the interview with Mrs. A., using the following symbols:
        ++     (very well),
        +      (well),
        +/-    (reasonably well)
        –      (moderate)
        - -    (poor)
    Critically reason your choice.

Figure 4. Individual analysis of the Case of Mrs. A

The important aspect of this lesson in terms of improving critical thinking skills is the careful questioning in the assignments guide (Figures 4 through 6). Here students are asked to think through the case and the interview, analyze and evaluate their own thinking processes (Figures 4 and 7), comparison with a colleague's thinking process (Figure 5), engage in collaborative critical thinking to reach consensus on the diagnoses (Figure 6), and evaluate the logical strength of the thinking process through the identification of fallacies (Figure 7).

The assignments guide the critical thinking process, step by step. In each case the students are asked to draw inferences (make diagnoses) based on their assessment of the case data and then to evaluate those inferences. We often ask the students to provide a quality rating or some other type of categorical rating using a 4 or 5 point scale. Sometimes these are peer evaluations and sometimes they are self-evaluations. This rating provides a point for later discussion, but it is not the completion of the reasoning process. In addition they are asked many times to provide the bases for these clinical judgements and ratings. We use a phrase in Dutch that would be translated "Critically reason your choice." which is the same as asking them to explain their chosen response. We expect them to be fair-minded and thorough in their critique of self and colleague.

## 2. Exchange of information.

Give the answers with elaboration to the questions 1a to 1e) to your colleague and receive from your colleague his/her elaboration (critique). Carefully read the elaboration of your colleague, make notes, and indicate what things are not clear. First discuss what was not clear. Then write down with your colleague the answers to the following questions.

> 2a- Where do your colleague's answers (1 to 1e) differ from your own answers? Give your view on your colleague's interpretation. Indicate if, compared to your own interpretation, your colleague's interpretation was more correct or less correct in arriving at the diagnoses.

> 2b- If there are differences: What according to both of you are the reasons underlying these differences? If there are significant differences in the diagnoses made by more nurses who have had a conversation with the same patient, we use the term inter-assessor variation. Write down examples of inter-assessor variation that arose during your discussion.

> 2c- Could inter-assessor variation also have any advantages? (For example, multidisciplinary consultation). Does inter-assessor have any disadvantages for the patient? If not, why not, if yes, why? Substantiate your opinion.

> 2d- What, in your opinion, are the possibilities to reduce the inter-assessor variation?

> 2e- Give a mark for the work of your colleague, using the following symbols:
> ```
> ++      (very good)
> +       (good)
> +/-     (reasonable)
> –       (moderate)
> - -     (poor)
> ```

This question will also be discussed during the plenary meeting afterwards. Try to be as critical as possible and to substantiate your opinion as carefully as possible.

## 3. Try to reach a consensus on the diagnoses made

> 3a- Write down the consensus diagnoses

> 3b- Write down on what points you reached a consensus and why this was so. (Also write down any differences of opinion that arose during the discussion).

Figure 5. Comparative Analyses of the Case of Mrs. A.

## 4. Analysis of the diagnostic reasoning

By completing assignments 1, 2 and 3 you have tried to identify as best you can the diagnosis of the patient. One form of reasoning begins with a major theory, generalization, fact, or premise that generates specific details and predictions. This is reasoning from the universal to the particular; that what is true of a class of things is true of each member of that class. It is called deductive because *"Deductive reasoning" can be defined as follows: if the facts in the premises are true, then the conclusion must be true.* However, we sometimes assume that generalizations are true when they might not be (Wilkinson, 2007).

Give on the basis of the consensus diagnoses two examples of deductive abduction by indicating:
1.
- knowledge rule:……………………..
- data:………………………..
- conclusion:………………………..
2.
- knowledge rule:……………………..
- data:………………………..
- conclusion:………………………..

4a- In the theory an explanation was given of "inductive reasoning." On the basis of the consensus diagnoses, give two examples of inductive reasoning. Motivate why your example is a case of inductive reasoning.

4b- Analyze the notes that you and your colleague wrote doing the above exercises, for evidence of logical fallacies. If you find evidence that you have committed one of these fallacies, which fallacy is it? Motivate why this is a fallacy.

4c- List a number of examples of the straw man fallacy. Describe any experiences of the straw man fallacy that resulted from the elaboration of the case.

4d- Assess the extent to which you use fallacies in conversations with fellow students, using the following symbols:
- ++ never
- +  rarely
- +/- sometimes
- -  often
- -- always

Motivate your choice. If your score is other than: ++, indicate why you use the fallacy. Describe briefly the disadvantages it may have for your patients in the clinical practice if you are not aware of your fallacious thinking.

4e- Earlier inventories show that nurses identify a lack of substantive knowledge and lack of time as the two main reasons for a fallacy to occur when diagnosing in practice. Do you agree with this? Why? Why not? Motivate your answer. Are there any other influencing factors?

**Figure 6: Critique of the Reasoning Process**

> **5 Evaluation**
> - Award yourself a mark from 1 to 10 about the quality of the diagnoses you have made and the arguments you have used.
> - Also award a mark to your colleague for the diagnoses he or she has made and the arguments used.
> - Give a mark for the consensus diagnoses.
>
> Is there a difference between the three marks? Make a note of the reasons why there are, or why there are not.
>
> > 5a. Given the lesson's learning objectives, how meaningful did you find the assignments?
> > Use the following symbols in your answer:
> > - ++     very meaningful
> > - +     meaningful
> > - -     not meaningful enough
> > - --     completely useless
> >
> > Motivate your opinion.
>
> > 5b. To end with the adage: "Look before you leap"
> > Answer or give your opinion on the following statement:
> >
> > `A nurse who is expected to identify the problems of a patient in preparing to provide nursing care owes it to the patient to develop diagnostic reasoning skills and should be aware of his or her own potential to commit fallacies.´
> >
> > - ++     agree strongly
> > - +     agree
> > - -     disagree
> > - --     disagree strongly
> >
> > Critically reason your opinion.

**Figure 7: Final self evaluation**

## How we evaluate the lesson

All students are asked to make notes during assignments 1 to 5. That includes writing down their individually found answers to each question and the results of discussions with their fellow student (in pairs). These notes are handed in to the teacher together with their (individually) written summary of the plenary discussion after assignment 5. In this summary, the student are asked to analyze if (and if so in what way) their answers to the questions in assignments 1 through 5 have changed as a result of the plenary discussion.

All students receive written feedback from the teacher and we've worked to make our feedback consistent across all the members of the teaching professor group. We've developed our consensus list of diagnoses which we have included here and which we use to check the conclusions students reach about the case (See Figure 8). We also examine their comments carefully for evidence of their meeting our learning objectives for critical reasoning.

| | |
|---|---|
| Diagnoses (actual physical): | 1) Tiredness.<br>2) Health negligence **OR** Ineffective therapy management; |
| Diagnosis (actual psycho-social): | Social isolation. |
| Diagnosis (potential physical): | Risk of injury in event of emotional disturbances, deteriorated eyesight and hypoglycaemia. |
| Diagnosis (potential psycho-social): with divorce. Missing loved ones. | Anticipating grief; coping |

**Figure 8: Answer key: Correct nursing diagnoses in diagnostic labels in the aforementioned case:**

**Student feedback on this lesson**

Students find this case-oriented, guided critical reasoning method, enjoyable to use. Nevertheless, generally spoken, it is not easy for the most of them. Nurses need conceptual understanding of the reasoning process itself. This tutorial balances conceptual and practical aspects, and that is what students like the most about this method. In a short time students have the experience that critical reasoning is the heart of nursing. Students like to participate in this tutorial because they see directly the progress they make.

One of the students noted down in an evaluation: *"Now I can see that there is a connection between rather boring theories about critical reasoning, deduction and induction and what you can do with it when you can use and implement these theories in everyday practice on the ward."*

Another student claimed: *"It is sometimes frustrating because the truth is not always what you intuitively think it is. It was one of my traps in thinking I wasn't aware of. I now experienced that reasoning skills are important. I need these skills before I can note down accurate diagnoses and interventions."*

Another student wrote this note: *"Seeking the truth is one of the most important habits. And, I thought, I was good at truth-seeking. Now I've learned that in many cases I can look further than I did before. I think I have to, because it benefits the patient in many ways."*

## Literature / References:

Carpenito, L.J. The NANDA definition of nursing diagnoses. In: Caroll Johnson, R.M. (Ed.) *Classifications of Nursing Diagnoses, Proceedings of Ninth Conference*, Philadelphia, J.B. Lippincott Company., 1991.

Gordon, M. *Nursing Diagnosis: Process and Application.* St. Louis: Mosby, 1994.

Lunney, M. (1992). Development of Written Case Studies as Simulations of Diagnoses in Nursing, *Nursing Diagnoses*, 3, 23-29.

Lunney, M. 2003, Critical Thinking and Accuracy of Nursing Diagnoses, *Nursing Diagnosis*, 6(1), 9-15.

NANDA, *Nanda Nursing Diagnoses: definitions & classification 2003-2004*, North American Nursing Diagnosis Association, NANDA International, Philadelphia, 2003.

Wilkinson, J..M., *Nursing Process and Critical Thinking*, Pearson Prentice Hall Health, New Jersey., 2007.

# Promoting Cognitive and Metacognitive Thinking Skills by Reflecting with Self-Regulated Learning Prompts

## *RuthAnne Kuiper*

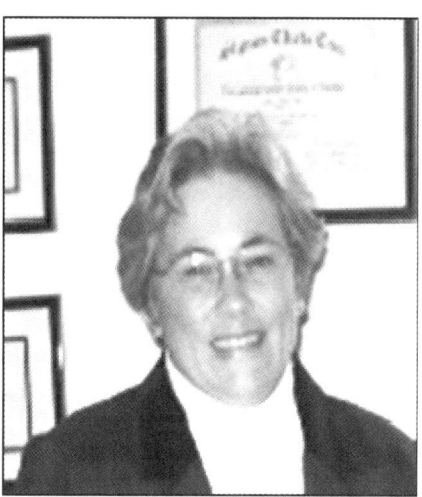

*Dr. RuthAnne Kuiper is an Associate Professor in the School of Nursing at the University of North Carolina, Wilmington in North Carolina, USA. She is a clinical specialist in cardiopulmonary nursing and focuses her teaching and research on the health issues of adults with critical illnesses. Her long term interest in clinical reasoning, specifically fostering cognitive and metacognitive thinking at all levels of nursing practice, has been a well matched asset for training Masters level nurse clinicians.*

*This exercise uses journaling to support self-regulatory learning. Students and clinical interns are practiced in the art of situational analysis and reflective self-evaluation. The goal of the exercise is to develop the habit of meta-cognitively monitoring one's thinking process, a vital attribute of the accomplished critical thinker. A number of other published papers by Dr Kuiper are mentioned in the reference list.*

### Clinical instruction session and students

This thinking exercise was developed as a part of a clinical internship for newly graduated registered nurses, and has since been used for new hires in a perioperative orientation program, and with undergraduate junior and senior level nursing students. My application of the technique to medical surgical nursing could easily be adapted to any program or practicing clinician group in the health sciences.

### The goal of the clinical instruction session

The complexity of any clinical scenario may overwhelm the student or novice clinician who is learning to practice in the health sciences. This exercise focuses on fostering growth in metacognition, a key critical thinking skill necessary for clinical reasoning and practicing the skills of reflection as a learning strategy (Brookfield, 1987; Facione, 1990). In developing this exercise I had several goals in mind. First, I wanted to apply what I knew of self-regulated learning strategies to optimally influence novice clinician's cognitive processes during a time when they were learning new skills in the clinical setting. Second, I wanted the exercise to promote recall and reflective thinking to maximize learning gained through practice experience. Finally I wanted to promote critical thinking skill acquisition. All of my goals could be met through the use of a structured self-regulated journaling exercise where the prompts serve to create habits of thinking that foster efficient and effective problem solving. These prompts can be used with individuals, or as a guide for focused debriefing with a group of students or clinicians.

## Learning objectives

Student interns (or novice clinicians) who participate in this reflective journal exercise will meet the following learning objectives:

- By reflectively examining their sense of self-efficacy, goals, knowledge sources and affective reactions, they will be able to self-evaluate, organize, monitor and correct their thinking processes.

- By observing their performance, thoughts and reactions, they will be able to motivate themselves to improve learning and self-efficacy and self-monitor their behaviors toward the attainment of a goal.

- Gain the ability to structure the contextual environment and social interaction as a background for metacognitive reflection and the monitoring of other critical thinking skills.

## Journaling Exercise

Optimal benefit from the journal prompts requires an introduction to Self-Regulated Learning Theory and, so I spend a bit of class time discussing this. A full discussion of this model of adult learning is published elsewhere (Kuiper & Hooks, 2004). Figure 1 shows its related concepts and sub-concepts. While one need not necessarily think of the model when writing responses to prompts, understanding the foundation for the prompts assists in attaining more complete responses. It is also crucial to remind the student interns that their responses will not be evaluated for a grade so that they will record thoughts that are spontaneous and uninhibited. I recommend that they do this self-regulated reflection exercise following a clinical experience, recording their responses either in writing or on audio-tape. The focus of the clinical situation can vary, but the reflective journaling should be done as close to the experience as possible to optimize the accuracy of the recall.

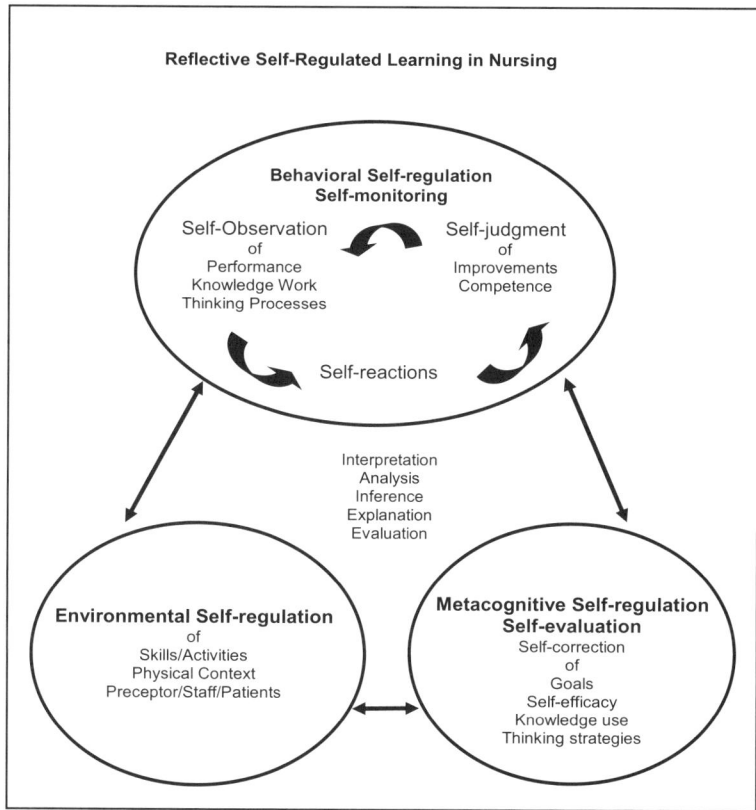

Figure 1: Reflective Self Regulation in Nursing

Kuiper, R. A. (2002) Enhancing metacognition through the reflective use of self-regulated learning strategies. *The Journal of Continuing Education in Nursing*, 33(2), 78-87. Reprinted here with permission.

In the critical thinking literature, metacognitive reflection involves 'thinking about your thinking.' In the middle of the model are the words Interpretation,

Analysis, Inference, Explanation and Evaluation. These are the five critical thinking skills identified by the American Philosophical Association's Delphi Study (Facione, 1990). The descriptions of these skills were derived from the consensus opinion of a multidisciplinary group of scholars. They continue to serve us today as common language for the reasoning skills needed to carry out a reflective self-regulatory exercise to assess progress toward a goal, in this case the progress toward competent clinical practice.

Journaling alone will not necessarily result in forming reasoning habits that involve critical thinking. What is needed are prompts that require the clinician to engage in a thinking process involving interpretation, analysis, inference-making, and self evaluation using the clinical experience as its information base,

**How I introduce this exercise**

Clinical interns are encouraged to journal after each clinical experience, and at a minimum, one additional time each week, thinking about that week's clinical experiences. I make the self regulated learning prompts and instructions for carrying out the exercise available in both hard copy and as an electronic e-mail attachment (Figure 2). I also stress that this is an individual metacognitive exercise, not group work and discourage student interns from sharing their work with other interns or with the clinical staff. Sharing thoughts leads to the incorporation of others' perspectives and negates the purpose of the exercise.

I've found that the journaling exercise should continue for a minimum of at least 5 to 6 weeks to develop a consistent behavior of reflective thought and to carry the intern past the period of clinical unit orientation. The work product is a series of journal entries or a "reflective log" of narratives that correspond to the clinical week assignments.

**Instructions:**

Please respond to each of the prompts as you reflect on your clinical experiences. Reflect on the thinking processes you used in clinical this week. Be sure to fully explain your responses.

1. The problems I encountered in clinical were...
    I think I solved them by...
    When I had difficulty I....
2. When I think about my feelings during the clinical experience, I would describe them as...
    and I handled them by...
3. When I try to remember or understand important facts to solve a problem, I....
4. As I look back, I could have spent:
    More time on....
    Less time on....

**Reflect on the environmental circumstances you encountered in clinical this week.**

5. When I prepare to carry out nursing activities on the clinical unit, I....
6. When I think about particular distractions on the clinical unit, I...
7. When I work with others or need help in the clinical area, I....

**Reflect on your behaviors and reactions to the clinical experiences this week. Be sure to give reasons for your self evaluation. Think about examples of your actual thoughts and behaviors and try to write a thoughtful explanation as you do these reflective exercises.**

8. My impression my performance in clinical this week was that I....
9. I make sure I complete my clinical assignment by....
    and if I need to make changes, I....
10. Reaction to clinical experiences:
    My reaction to what I liked about the clinical experiences this week was....
11. My reaction to what I did not like about the clinical experiences this week was....

When you have finished journaling, send your journal to your clinical instructor/preceptor for feedback. Don't forget to put your name on the work. Include a research article that you retrieved and read as a part of better understanding your clinical experience and related best practices. Be sure to discuss how the research article relates to your journal comments.

**Figure 2: Self-regulation Learning Prompts for Reflection on Clinical Experiences**

Adapted from Kuiper, R. A. (2000). A new direction for cognitive development in nursing to prepare the practitioners of the future. *Nursing Leadership Forum*, 4(4), 116-124.

## Evaluation and Feedback

While there is no grade attached to this exercise, faculty are eager for the student to reflect in ways that tap the cognitive and metacognitive thinking skills that will support and strengthen clinical reasoning, build domain specific knowledge stored in long term memory, and create a habitual way of thinking that leads to effective and efficient clinical decision making. Many individuals require a bit of formative feedback and guidance for this to happen. Giving feedback on the specific concepts in the model will reinforce the use of metacognitive thinking and encourage those activities that are missing. This is important since more complete use of the model results in higher-order thinking (causal and comparative statements) and deeper levels of reflection.

The evaluation guide for the self-regulation learning prompts (Figure 3) assists faculty in determining the depth of responses and helps them observe changes in an individual's journaling over time. Comments show interns the areas where deeper levels of reflection and thought are possible for continued growth. One can also look for evidence of the critical thinking embedded in the narrative responses (analysis, explanation, evaluation, interpretation, inference). Verb tense evaluation gives clues as to whether the student draws on past experiences and/or can plan future activities. Script analysis can be used to identify the common/uncommon themes reflected by this group, this student, or in a particular clinical experience.

Table 1 below provides some examples of how I evaluate journal responses. The comments in the column headed 'Example' are taken directly from a student's journal. Common themes of reflective thinking can be extracted and trended over time to show growth and change in student thinking. Critical thinking skills embedded in the responses can also be evaluated and exposed for students to be able to see their proficiency and areas for improvement, Table 2.

I.  **Metacognitive Self-Evaluation** (self-corrective thinking processes)
    Identify reference to or evidence of:
    a.  goals mentioned in relation to desired changes…
    b.  knowledge work, resources to improve knowledge…
    c.  affect such as personal emotional responses (happy, sad, satisfied, frightened, anxious)…
    d.  self-efficacy to the extent that they were capable/incapable of completing perceived tasks, challenges…

II. **Behavioral Self-Monitoring**
    Identify reference to or evidence of:
    a.  self-observations of performance, knowledge work, thinking processes…
    b.  self-reactions of general environment, circumstances…
    c.  self-judgments of improvements, competence…

III. **Environmental Self-Regulation**
    Identify reference to or evidence of:
    a.  environmental circumstances associated with skills, activities, physical context…
    b.  persons such as peers, colleagues, health care team, patients, families…

IV. **Embedded Critical Thinking Skills**
    Identify reference to or evidence of:
    a.  Analysis and explanation of affective reactions to the clinical experience
    b.  Fair-minded inferences about performance of practice skills and self efficacy
    c.  Evaluation of performance using relevant criteria
    d.  Comprehensive analysis of problems
    e.  Exploration and analysis of potential solutions
    f.  Reason giving for decisions made in the practice setting

**Figure 3: Evaluation Guide for Self-regulation Learning Prompt Responses**

Table 1: Embedded Reflective Thinking Themes

| REFLECTIVE THINKING THEMES | EXAMPLE |
|---|---|
| Observations of knowledge work | Next week I will read more in preparation for clinical. <br><br> I organize in my mind the information I need for the clinical record in order of importance. |
| Observations of thinking strategies | I will think of possible solutions and consult with a preceptor or experienced nurse. <br><br> I focus on what I should be doing. |
| Judgments of self-improvement | I am beginning to learn a little regarding diabetes complications. <br><br> I have been thinking how far I have come. |
| Judgments of self-competence | I was disorganized this past week. I feel I need to be more assertive and voice my learning needs to others. |
| Judgments of resources | I worked with my preceptor and he was a very good teacher. He was patient and answered all my questions. <br><br> I have the necessary resources. |
| Judgments of social interactions | Working with others is very important, I always try to be a team player. <br><br> Has been pleasant and helpful, however, I wish I could have been given more independence. |
| Self-reactions | I feel slightly more relaxed in the clinical area. <br><br> I feel a bit overwhelmed. |
| Self-correction strategies | Try to have a better attitude. <br><br> I will try to start fresh. <br><br> I will try to be more familiar with the types of cases we get on this unit. |

## Table 2: Embedded Critical Thinking Skills

| SKILL | EXAMPLE |
|---|---|
| Analysis | Everyone else was having anxiety as well, and I wasn't doing any worse then they were.<br><br>I was able to fill out paper work fairly well. |
| Inference<br>Analysis<br>Evaluation | I wish the staff would stop making me feel stupid, with time I will get it. I would like to see them function in other clinical areas.<br><br>Some staff have not been helpful, they forgot what it is like to start over. |
| Evaluation | I felt like I finally took care of a case on my own.<br><br>I survived five admissions with no problems. |
| Explanation | I feel with time I will be able to focus past distractions because....<br><br>I am optimistic about my ability to conquer adversity because..... |
| Analysis<br>Interpretation | Read about the medical diagnoses and try to keep an upbeat attitude.<br><br>I deliberately kept my goals simple and use them as a foundation for improving. |

## Final comments on this thinking exercise

This self-regulation reflection exercise guides the multidimensional consideration of every aspect of a situation. It trains interns to become more metacognitive in their clinical reasoning in practice on a daily basis. It encourages the monitoring of thinking processes, reactions, and an attention to the environment. Those who practice this exercise become more metacognitive about how they make judgments and revise plans or approaches. By using self-regulated learning strategies, clinicians can reflect on their performance and build on experiences more efficiently, thus promoting competent practice.

## References

Brookfield, S.D. *Developing critical thinkers: Challenging adults to explore alternative ways of thinking and acting.* San Francisco, CA: Jossey Bass, 1987.

Facione, PA, (1990). "The Delphi Report Executive Summary" *ERIC*, ED 315423. Montclair, NJ: Montclair State University Center for Critical Thinking. And Millbrae, CA: The California Academic Press. 1-22.Kuiper, R. A. (2000). A new direction for cognitive development in nursing to prepare the practitioners of the future. *Nursing Leadership Forum*, 4(4), 116-124.

Kautz, D. D., Kuiper, R. A., & Pesut, D. J. (2005). Promoting clinical reasoning in undergraduate nursing students: Application and evaluation of the Outcome Present State Test (OPT) Model of clinical reasoning. *International Journal of Nursing Education Scholarship*, 12(1). http://www.bepress.com/ijnes/vol12/iss1/art1

Kautz, D. D., Kuiper, R. A., Pesut, D. J., & Williams, R. L. (2006). Unveiling the use of NANDA, NIC, and NOC (NNN) Language with the Outcome-Present State Test Model of Clinical Reasoning, *International Journal of Nursing Terminologies and Classifications*, 17(3). 129-138.

Kuiper, R. A. (2002). Enhancing metacognition through the reflective use of self-regulated learning strategies. *The Journal of Continuing Education in Nursing*, 33(2), 78-87.

Kuiper, R. A. (2004). Nursing reflections from journaling during a perioperative internship. *AORN*, 79(1), 195-218.

Kuiper, R. A. (2005). Self-regulated Learning during a Clinical Preceptorship: The Reflections of Senior Baccalaureate Nursing Students, *Nursing Education Perspectives*, 26(6). 351-356.

Kuiper, R. A. & Hooks R. (2004). An Examination of the Impact of Self-regulated Learning Strategies on Practicing Nurses. *On Line Journal of Sigma Theta Tau International.* http://www/nursingsociety.org/education/SQ0002/sq0002_index.html.

Kuiper, R. A. & Pesut, D. J. (2004). Promoting cognitive and metacognitive reflective clinical reasoning skills in nursing practice: self-regulated learning theory. *Journal of Advanced Nursing*, 45(4), 381-391.

# Prioritizing Nursing Assessments and Care

## *Susan A. Sandstrom*

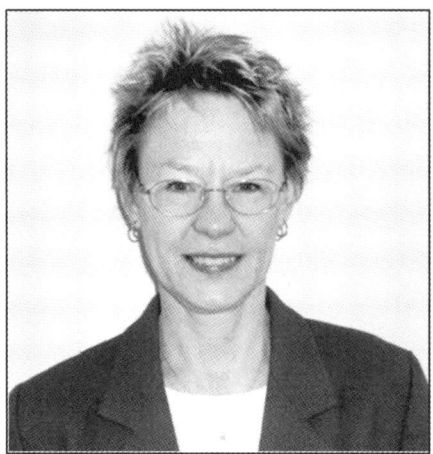

*Susan Sandstrom is an Associate Professor of Nursing in the School of Health Professions at the College of Saint Mary, an all women's Catholic college in Omaha Nebraska, United States. Her areas of clinical expertise include intensive and coronary units and medical-surgical nursing and she has taught medical-surgical nursing for more than 20 years. Professor Sandstrom brings us a lesson in the application of theoretical models.*

*We particularly like this chapter because of the evolving client scenario and the invitation to students to think in groups about what new patient assessment data they require and why. Professor Sandstrom's description of how she teaches this lesson suggests that she is an inspirational teacher who has a bit of a gift for theatre as well. Her focus on teaching pedagogy is also shared in a paper she wrote on the use of case studies to teach health science content cited at the end of this chapter.*

### An overview of the class exercise and my goal for the session

The exercise has two parts, the first involving a determination of needed interventions for a client described in a scenario, and the second involving a discussion of their chosen interventions. In the first part of the exercise students are asked to discuss symptomatology and interventions that could affect the client's condition. The critical thinking skills emphasized in the first part of this exercise are: 1) inference, 2) interpretation, 3) analysis, and 4) evaluation. In the final discussion of the results of their actions in the scenario, the critical thinking skills of explanation and self-regulation are also utilized.

I ask students to discuss their thinking process with their peers for two reasons. First, the work of health science practitioners is a collaborative effort and this peer conversation sets the expectation that as clinicians they will serve clients better through collaborative analysis of client problems and plans of intervention. Second, discussing their thinking process with a peer forces students to do a more careful analysis and interpretation of the client's situation. They realize that they may be asked by a peer to explain their client assessment.

My goal for student learning in this experience is for students to use their clinical reasoning and critical thinking skills while applying their knowledge of assessment to determine priority actions to best help the client.

**Learning objectives:**

After each learning objective I have listed one or more critical thinking skills that are emphasized when students work to meet the objective (see parentheses)

Students who participate in this experience will be able to:

1. Identify the priority needs of the client from the information given. (analysis).
2. Seek out additional information from the client and family members needed for your assessment. (inference).
3. Clarify the meaning of and identify the significance of the assessments in this situation. (interpretation, inference and explanation).
4. Examine the ideas peers present to help this client. (evaluation)
5. Infer (plan) the best course of action for this client (inference).
6. Justify the planned course of action with rationale. (inference, explanation and evaluation).
7. Self-examine the decisions made related to the results of those decisions for this client (evaluation).

**Class session and students:**

I teach this class session during a clinical day in the beginning of the final course in an Associate degree nursing program. In many ways it is a capstone course where students need to demonstrate competence in patient assessment and outline a plan of care. The course, and particularly this class exercise, requires students to apply assessment skills and previous learning of health science content knowledge to develop the best course of action for the patient. Before entering this class, students have had coursework in assessment, cardiac dysfunction and material on teaching and learning concepts.

## The actual material used for class session:

This lesson requires me to prepare in advance a hypothetical client case. The case begins as a scenario describing the first encounter between the nurse and the client. This type of scenario works well because it fits with the goal of the exercise which is to call forth the student's client assessment skills. This example lesson is from a class of nursing students but the exercise would work just as well in a staff development workshop. The scenario is necessarily brief and offers the details about the client that a nurse might readily observe from report and from initial visual encounter of the patient. Figure one below is an example of a scenario I might use for this exercise.

> You have been assigned a newly admitted client with a diagnosis of Trigeminal Neuralgia. Mr. Mannelli is a 66 year old insurance salesman who was admitted at 10:00 p.m. the previous evening. His vital signs on admission were: T $98^4$; P 100; R 20; BP 110/60 sitting. He is 6 ft tall and weighs 270 lbs. You are making your initial rounds at 8:30 a.m. as report lasted longer than usual. When you walk into Mr. Mannelli's room to make your initial assessment, Mr. Mannelli's wife and daughter are also in the room. You sense that something isn't quite right with Mr. Mannelli. What would you do in order of priority? Your instructor will supply you with any additional data you request. (Assessments and Data follow on faculty data sheet.)

**Figure 1 The scenario of Mr. Mannelli's case:**

I also prepare in advance a data sheet that corresponds with the client scenario that I have planned for the session. On the data sheet I record more information about the client in the scenario so that I am readily able to provide this information to the students in response to their comments and questions about the client in the scenario. Figure 2 below is an example data sheet that corresponds with the Scenario in Figure 1. The case must be at the level of difficulty appropriate for the class. In the example case below the students are relative novices in a nursing education program.

While I might easily provide a hypothetical case without pre-planning the details, having them in hand assures consistency with an authentic clinical case. And more importantly it frees me to attend to the kinds of questions and clinical interpretations being made by the students participating in the session. I can put my attention to analyzing their responses and asking them to explain their requests for client assessment data. "What assumption is behind your request for data about this client's respiratory status?"

| Assessment | Data |
|---|---|
| Respiratory Status | Dyspnea, increased resp. rate 32/min shallow |
| Lung sounds | Rales and rhonchi heard without a stethoscope |
| Color | Cyanotic, diaphoretic |
| Tissue perfusion | Poor return from extremities, cold and cyanotic extremities, pitting edema |
| Mental status | Short attention span, irritable, appears anxious |
| Vital signs | P 140; R 32; BP 90/50 |
| Intake/Output | Increase in weight last month of 15 lbs (may ask family for this information) Urine output – unknown, not catheterized; family doesn't think he's voided since admission |
| Abdomen | Noticeable ascities |
| Hepatic status | Enlarged liver – tender to palpation |
| Venous status | Distended jugular veins at 45 degree angle |
| Vital signs | P 150; R 30; BP 80/30 |
| Current orders | Demerol 50 mg prn pain; up and about as tolerated; low Na+, low fat diet; home meds |
| History (from family) | Long history of congestive heart failure. Daughter is a nurse and an excellent resource. Home meds: Capoten (ace inhibitor), Lasix (diuretic), Lanoxin (inotrope), Coreg (Beta blocker) |

Figure 2: Data sheet for Mr. Mannelli's case

## Teaching the lesson

The students can either receive a written client scenario or it can be read to them, as if they were receiving report on this new client. In either case they are expected to seek all relevant assessment data then decide what to do. No client assessment information is provided to the students unless they ask for it. If the students decide to call the physician, talk to the family or to the client, I play the part of these people and give their responses. The actual material on my data sheet (Figure 2) only shows how the client declines if nothing is done and can even progress to death. If the students continue to falter in developing a complete assessment of the client, I heat up the symptoms and add to the pressure to achieve a complete client assessment and plan of action. But as the students make appropriate decisions, I allow the client to improve. The scenario should unfold as closely as possible to an actual practice situation.

This exercise is not meant for students to focus on making new diagnoses, but rather to focus on interpreting what is happening with their client and to act on that assessment even when these events are not related to the admitting medical diagnosis. It is meant to help them work together, use their assessment skills, prioritize their assessments, and to plan care that the client actually needs, not based only on the admitting diagnosis. The students are able to utilize textbooks or other resources to look up questions they have about the client's condition, but the scenario progresses rapidly (within 10 minutes) and the client deteriorates if the students do not rapidly act on the information they have.

## What I expect from class participants

This exercise could easily be done in a large class or conference environment if the professor sets the expectation with the group that each person will work independently first to think through the task of the assessment before the new assessment data is revealed. But it is also easily run with a small group of students (8-10), When I use it in small groups, I expect every student to participate in this exercise, and in the small group there is more likely participation even when they are unsure if they are correct or not. This allows learning from their peers to occur. Small group exercises do require some classroom management to be sure that the session is not dominated by only one or two students.

If there is a student in the group who usually takes over discussions, use a strategy of requiring the students to go around the group listening to each student offer an analysis and interpretation of the case before any student offers a decision about what assessment data should be requested; what information should be reported to the physician; or what specific orders should be requested from the physician. This not only assures that each student participates, but also practices the expectation of providing clear descriptions of their assumptions about the client (the critical thinking skills of interpretation and inference). They will also more fully develop rationale for the client assessment data they will soon request from me.

In this scenario, I have intentionally set up the situation where this client's admitting medical diagnosis has nothing to do with his current condition. I want students to discover this through their analysis of the early information provided as a response to their requests for information about Mr. Manelli. In addition, this strategy provides me more than ample opportunity to anecdotally assess my student's critical thinking disposition as a clinical team. The willingness to engage new problems is essential to the skilled critical thinker. Needing to know what is happening when things are different than expected is a demonstration of the critical thinking disposition of inquisitiveness and analyticity.

Pursuing the novel problem even when it does not fit a current problem frame engages the critical thinking dispositions of truth seeking, analyticity, and the cognitive maturity in prioritizing the data. Thinking through the client assessment until a complete picture of the case is achieved demonstrates systematicity. This terminology about critical thinking dispositions comes from the American Philosophical Association study on critical thinking referenced at the end of this chapter.

Also in the interest of client safely, I expect students to do priority assessments for all clients where they "sense that something isn't quite right." These assessments should begin with airway, breathing and circulation. In my experience using this exercise, students often flounder a little and then successfully focus in on the respiratory and cardiac systems as a guide to their assessments. Knowledge of the congestive heart failure disease process is part of their knowledge base from a previous course, so they should be familiar with the signs and symptoms of this disease process and be able to recognize this pattern in their assessment. As with every effective classroom or staff development exercise, the thinking task must be well chosen to be within the knowledge base of the student or staff person. Otherwise the assessment of inability to think well about a patient assessment might be inaccurate and really only attributable to a lack of knowledge of the disease process involved.

**The student work product**

I use this exercise early in the course and it is not attached to a specific written course assignment. My assessment of the student's ability to use critical thinking skills in this clinical situation is done during their discussion. Those faculty who are less practiced at listening for evidence of critical thinking skills should prepare a short rubric that reminds the listener of the observable evidence of displayed critical thinking skill as this might appear in the assignment, or you might consider using the Holistic Critical Thinking Scoring Rubric (HCTSR), a free download on the website: www.InsightAssessment.com/hctsr.html when the purpose of use is educational assessment.[3]

For those who would like to link this exercise to a written assignment, it can be connected to a resultant nursing process plan that the students turn in for the client. That written work is based on the same process that they used in finding out more about the situation: gathering available data, seeking out further information, analyzing the information to determine the client's priority need, planning client care, justifying the plan with the rationale for nursing actions planned, and evaluating the outcome or the client's response to care. To evaluate the critical thinking that was used in the development of the process plan, you might add a column that requests the student or clinician to document the assumption that they made when seeking the assessment data. If done well this request will provide some evidence of the critical thinking skills of analysis, inference and explanation.

### Feedback from the students

Students of all levels typically like this class exercise. It reminds them that they need to be aware of not only what their client's medical diagnosis is but also the current physical assessment of what is happening now with their client and the client's history. It also reminds them of the benefits of using more than one source of data to provide the best care for their client. Their eager participation in the peer thinking exercise also demonstrates that they enjoy the opportunity to practice thinking skills in this type of context.

### References

*American Philosophical Association Delphi Research Report,* ERIC Document Number: ED 315 423. Or download the executive summary from The California Academic Press. http://www.insightassessment.com/dex.html

Sandstrom, S. (2006). Use of Case Studies to Teach Diabetes and Other Chronic Illnesses to Nursing Students. *Journal of Nursing Education*, 45(6), 229-232

---

[3] Preprinted with instructions for use in the mini-chapter on the HCTST by Peter Facione

# Teaching Critical Thinking in Medicine: A Journey Back to the Future

## *Milos Jenicek*

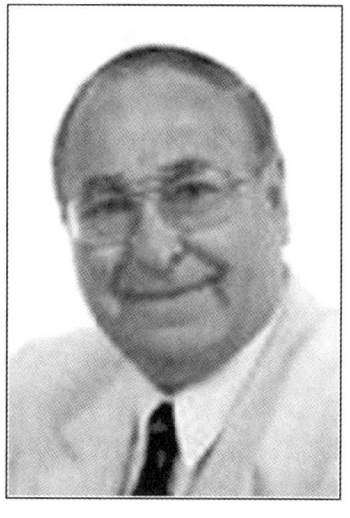

*Dr. Jenicek is a Professor in the Department of Clinical Epidemiology and Biostatistics, Michael de Groote School of Medicine, McMaster University, Hamilton, Ontario, Canada. He is also Professor Emeritus at the Université de Montréal and Adjunct Professor at McGill University, Montréal, Québec, Canada. He has been a visiting scholar in United States (Harvard, Johns Hopkins, Yale, UNC Chapel Hill and the Uniformed Services at Bethesda) Hong Kong, Singapore, Japan, South Korea, Portugal, Brazil, France and Switzerland, and a visiting professor to various universities and governments in France, Spain, Switzerland, Portugal, Morocco, Algeria, Czech Republic, Singapore, Korea, and Kuwait. We are very honored by Dr. Jenicek's contribution to this international volume.*

*Dr. Jenicek's publications have given the world its understanding of evidence based practice. You will hear more about several of them below, but we direct you to these famous texts: "Epidemiology. The Logic of Modern Medicine" (EPIMED International,1995, in Spanish 1996, in Japanese 1998); "Medical Casuistics. Proper Reporting of Clinical Cases" (in French, 1997); "Clinical Case Reporting in Evidence-Based Medicine" (Butterworth Heinemann,1999, 2$^{nd}$ Ed, 2001; in Italian 2001, in Korean 2002, in Japanese 2002; "Foundations of Evidence-Based Medicine" 2003; "Evidence-Based Practice. Logic and Critical Thinking in Medicine" (with D.L. Hitchcock, AMA Press, 2005); and "A Physician's Self-Paced Guide to Critical Thinking", AMA Press, 2006.*

*This chapter is an important orientation to the discovery of embedding critical thinking pedagogy into the content of a health sciences seminar session or bedside teaching opportunity. We expect that as you read this chapter, the critical thinking content in your own course offerings will become more and more transparent to you and to your students. The chapter follows a somewhat different format that the ones that follow. In his discussion, Dr. Jenicek offers us an opportunity to think about the historical influence of the critical thinking* movement on the teaching of medicine. His wisdom as an international scholar is apparent as he traces progress to date on our scholarly understanding of human reasoning and judgment and offers interesting reflections for future endeavors. The reference list at the end of this chapter will assist those who wish to aid the development of new science in this area. We particularly endorse his comment that the application of critical thinking to the procedures of clinical medicine, community health programs, bedside practice and health science researchers is the best way to attain relevant growth in clinical reasoning. He has also included the generous welcome that you to contact him at ***jenicekm@mcmaster.ca***

## Introduction

Is the teaching of critical thinking in medicine new? Yes and no, based on the author's learning, academic and professional experiences. Today, most North American medical schools and faculties have among their objectives to educate and train new health professionals as critical thinkers. In view of this objective, we wish to reflect here upon:

1. How we did this in the past;
2. What we are doing now; and
3. What should we strive to achieve in the future? What are the challenges of teaching critical thinking in medicine and how can we best face them in the years to come?

In the following pages I offer some possible answers to these questions.

Elements of modern critical thinking were taught in medicine for several generations under different labels and only more recently has critical thinking and its teaching emerged as an entity under its own name. Critical thinking *per se* has benefited from its contact with the basic sciences and almost all medical specialties and disciplines that support them like epidemiology, biostatistics and sociology on one side and philosophy on the other.

The past three or four generations of philosophers significantly enriched our understanding of informal logic, argument and argumentation as core elements in a wider spectrum of critical thinking in general. They advanced structured methodology and expanded uses and applications of critical thinking in an ever-growing number of domains of human life, biological sciences, social and other sciences and arts. The leap from ideas about critical thinking at the beginning of the past century[1,2] to contemporary informal logic[3], critical thinking[4] and its current vision[5,6] was enormous as can be seen from these very few examples and the illustrative references in this chapter. An even more considerable time span separates the classical forms of argumentation in ancient Greece[7] (the ubiquitous Aristotelian categorical syllogism, its *premises and conclusions* as its expression) and India[8] (Nyaya school, its *'demonstration'* through a *'proposition – reason – exemplification – application – conclusion'* complex) from logic and modern argument modeling[9] (involving *claim, grounds, backing, warrant, qualifier, rebuttals* as building blocks) and its applications[10]. Critical thinking appears now as important in the practice of medicine and the health sciences, in health science research, and in philosophy in medicine itself as are already medical ethics and epistemology of research. In these rapidly evolving times, fundamental tools are now available and new challenges and distinctions are developing.

Today, critical thinking in medicine and its teaching are at the crossroads of epidemiology, biostatistics, evidence-based medicine (EBM), and clinical teaching methodology. Which path should we choose? In discussing such a question here and in trying to find at least a partial answer, the reader should be aware that this is a personal reflection of a health professional and academic based mainly on a recent individual experience and acquired knowledge. It is unsupported so far by structured research, evaluation, integration and synthesis of various experiences with teaching critical thinking across medical academic and professional institutions. This will come only later. Medicine is not an exact science, but a biological one, bearing the inherent attributes of probability and uncertainty. Let us now take a closer look!

## 1. Past experience and contributions to critical thinking in medicine

In the search for the best possible description and understanding of disease and other health phenomena occurrence, biostatisticians and physicians played and are playing a major role in the development of the methodology required for the measurement, counting, quantification and classification of what was seen at the bedside and in the community. Thus, biometrics and clinimetrics were born.

In the search for the best possible proof and explanation of causes of disease occurrence and course, epidemiologists and biostatisticians refined the methodology of observational analytical studies. Clinical trialists adopted and further elaborated these causal thinking roots in the experimental method (clinical trials) as part of the general scientific method used in medicine. As they relate to critical thinking, these initiatives have so far been classified (in the spirit of this chapter) into two basic categories: causal thinking and logic of medicine, often within the larger framework of the philosophy of medicine.

In 'causal thinking,' John Stuart Mill's ideas about causes[11] were developed and adapted to the biological and social characteristics of medicine by physicians, dentists, biostatisticians and sociologists including C Bernard[12], AB Hill[13], J Jerushalmy and CE Palmer[14], RS Ludley and LB Lusted[15], AR Feinstein[16], B MacMahon and TF Pugh[17,18], experts involved in smoking and health evaluation[13,19], M Susser[20], C Buck[21], AS Evans[22], DL Weed[23], JM Elwood[24] S Greenland's[25] and KJ Rothman's[26] groups of authorities, to name just a few in somewhat chronological order (and with apologies to all the unnamed). We have reviewed, summarized, referenced and updated these contributions elsewhere[27].

In conjunction with causal considerations, various aspects of reasoning and logic in the framework of philosophy in medicine as a more distinct entity were proposed by LS King[28], EA Murphy[29], ED Pellegrino and DC Thomasma[30], HR Wulff et al.[31], CI Phillips' group[32], and also in fuzzy logic in medicine as originally advanced by LA Zadeh[33] and K Sadek-Zadeh[34]. In 1995, our '*Epidemiology. Logic of Modern Medicine*' [35] bore a rather cheeky subtitle referring to the logic behind epidemiology. A more distinct introductory coverage of logical aspects of evidence-based medicine[27] followed only in 2003. The relevance of argumentation in light of SE Toulmin's philosophy[9,10] was emphasized for medicine by R Horton[36] and presented even more forcefully later on by DL Hitchcock [37]. Fundamental notions of logic and critical thinking in medicine under this title[37] appeared in 2005, followed by a collection of suggested teaching and learning tools in a self-learning guide[38] in 2006.

## 2. General philosophy and strategies of teaching critical thinking in medicine today

To teach physicians critical thinking, we have to choose between two strategies: We can convey the message the way philosophers do for general studentship or we can apply critical thinking to the procedures followed by clinical medicine and community health programs practitioners at the bedside or in the community or to the procedures followed by health researchers in the performance of their scientific method and research protocols. The latter definitely appears more attractive and relevant for the action-oriented recipients of the message.

Reflecting on the second question of how we teach critical thinking in medicine today, I find it helpful to consider several distinct groups:

- Medical students and residents in various clinical specialties and in community and family medicine;
- Research oriented physicians;
- Clinical teachers and academic clinicians, 'teachers to be taught.'

## For all young physicians in training

From the currently available array of general critical thinking teaching methods[39,40] (classroom assessment techniques, cooperative learning strategies, case studies/discussion, using questions, conference style learning, writing assignments, dialogues, creating ambiguities in the group and solving them instantly), clinical cases studies at hospital floors, rounds and consults, case studies and medical information appraisal are essential training for undergraduates and graduates in medicine.

In medicine, related to the above mentioned techniques and strategies of teaching methods, two types of clinical teaching methods are currently often in use: Pimping and Socratic discourse. 'Pimping,'[41,42] in the field of medicine, refers to clinical practice teaching where persons in power ask questions (often irrelevant to the problem solution and/or unanswerable) of their junior colleagues with objectives ranging from knowledge acquisition to embarrassment, humiliation, and/or establishment of pecking order within the pimping/pimped group. So far, I have not met anyone who did not experience pimping during their medical training. Sometimes, pimping is intentional, sometimes, pimpers believe that this is the right way to lead others to desirable knowledge, attitudes or skills. Most of these are ignoring what we know as good pedagogy for teaching critical thinking today.

The **Socratic method**[43,44] which is a 'more participatory, focused, structured, goal oriented, and polite form of pimping' is also in use. Questions (directed uncertainty) are stated, answers to them are proposed, objectives and objections to the answer are explored, and answers are revised to stand up to all known relevant objections. Various Socratic – type questions[45] are used according to their nature (*clarification, probing assumptions - questions – reasons – evidence - implications and consequences, and revising viewpoints and perspectives*) in a clear direction in the problem understanding and solving process. To be effective, they should be systematic, directional, purpose driven, categorized, and not raised in a haphazard way. The Socratic method is therefore a cornerstone of teaching at the level of clinical physician. The Socratic method potentially falls short if the clinician fails to look closely enough at the argumentation being offered. Adding the more detailed learning of argumentation, argument construction (research projects) and reconstruction (critical appraisal of evidence and how the evidence is used in argumentation)[46-48] appears to be a necessary teaching and learning tool to be mastered and used by all academic physicians involved in classroom, laboratory or bedside teaching and research.

**For more experienced physicians (research oriented, clinical teachers and academic clinicians):**

In the spirit of the shortest definition of critical thinking[4], a *"reasonable reflective thinking that is focused on deciding what to believe or do"*, training oriented this way is perhaps optimal for medicine because it stresses two distinct entities that are inherent and vital to the profession: understanding a health problem (diagnosis, biological mechanisms, causes, history and prognosis) and decisions concerning how to solve it (exposure control, disease prevention and radical or conservative treatment, health promotion).

Health research applied to critical thinking and effective argumentations adds another necessary dimension to thinking critically in the health sciences. Scriven's and Paul's vision of critical thinking as *the intellectually disciplined process of actively and skillfully conceptualizing, applying, analyzing, synthesizing, and/or evaluating information gathered from, or generated by, observation, experience, reflection, reasoning, or communication, as a guide to belief and action*[49] is particularly attractive for any scientific method and research protocol practitioner given this definition's particular and almost explicit link to the scientific method.

Both of these concepts and definitions accurately reflect medical reasoning in understanding and actions.

**Examples of Teaching Critical Thinking in Medicine (TCTM)**

Besides *ad hoc* seminars and TCTM applied in a scattered manner across the health research methodology and other opportunities in fundamental and clinical epidemiology, two of our recent experiences are worth sharing. In both instances,[50,51] our goal was to introduce critical thinking, its objectives, relevance and illustrative applications to various health professionals, first in public health (*a*) and then in internal medicine (*b*). The Attachment at the end of this essay summarizes the statement of purpose, conceptual framework and content of those events.

**a. Critical thinking for public health professionals**

In the framework of continuing education, as directed and initiated by Dr. Freddie Asinor from the APHA a one-day workshop[50] (Institute CEI # 1003.0) entitled *"Evidence-Based Practice. Logic and Critical Thinking"* was given at the American Public Health Association's *APHA 133rd Annual Conference* in Philadelphia, December 2005. Physicians, public health nurses and others participated. Dr. David L. Hitchcock was my co-presenter at this event.

Let me take a moment to talk about Dr. Hitchcock who has a lifelong experience in graduate and undergraduate teaching of critical thinking. David is Professor of Philosophy at the McMaster University, and the author of *"Critical Thinking: A Guide to Evaluating Information."* He guided my writing of two chapters on logic and critical thinking in the book *Foundations of Evidence Based Medicine*.[27] This remarkable partnership and exceptional mutual understanding lead to a wonderful friendship and a future collaboration in the monograph entitled *Evidence-Based Practice. Logic and Critical Thinking in Medicine.*[37]

The purpose of the workshop was to offer participants an overview of the principles and methods of modern informal logic and critical thinking as used and required for effective formulation of public health programs and policies, priority setting, implementation, analysis and evaluation. The learning objectives were the following: In terms of attitudes, participants should come to realize that the production of the best evidence for effective public health decision making is not enough if it is not coupled and accompanied by the most rational and effective uses of the best evidence. In terms of knowledge, participants were lead to acquire a basic understanding of thinking critically about health problems and making decisions about them. In terms of skills, participants most importantly acquired the ability to apply the principles and techniques of logic and critical thinking to health problems under their jurisdiction, putting into practice the essential building blocks of modern argumentation and linking them in such a way to arrive at the best claims, proposals, and conclusions in the public health domain.

Teaching methods during the workshop included the identification of the participants' own needs and interests and expectations, small group discussions, and an analysis of cases like the Katrina public health disaster (DL Hitchcock) and one public health program evaluation article (M. Jenicek). On this occasion I asked participants to evaluate the paper entitled, "Effectiveness of school programs in preventing childhood obesity." by Veugelers and Fitzgerald.[78] The participants were asked to analyze the case and the program evaluation to identify and criticize the arguments being made by each. Both were used as illustrations of how arguments may and should be constructed and reconstructed for the benefit of health professionals in their understanding and decision-making.

As part of the teaching materials, the American Public Health Association has provided our own textbook, *Evidence-Based Practice. Logic and Critical Thinking in Medicine (2005)*[37] to each of the participants. In addition, we developed and distributed two new interactive exercises to each participant (with solutions provided only after the discussion and the analysis of both cases made first by small groups or couples of participants.) The solutions have been handed to participants in written (answers to questions related to Katrina disaster, as well as handwritten comments added into the original AJPH paper.

Prior to the workshop, we had invited participants to send us suggestions about which health problems would be of most interest to them in order to make the program even more relevant and tailored to their needs. Surprisingly, none of the participants brought or sent in advance any health problems to be discussed in the workshop. Nonetheless the workshop appeared to offer participants effective learning opportunities. The evaluation of our workshop presentation was formative, based on the subjective assessment by each participant. On a scale from one to five (one being poor and five being excellent), we were evaluated above 4 points for objectives, content, and presentation style, endorsing the value of the session. Only a lack of enough time and the wish that our health problems could have been distributed in advance were voiced as suggestions for improvement. In our own evaluation of the session, we noted a persistent confusion between critical appraisals of evidence as already rooted in evidence-based public health and critical thinking about the health problem supported by already appraised best evidence. We clarified this point again later in a special review and position paper[45].

**b. Critical thinking for internists**

On October 18th and 19th, 2006, the Department of Medicine of the University of Calgary, Alberta and the Alberta Medical Association (Physician and Family Support Program) organized and sponsored a series of seminars for residents, internists and academic staff in internal medicine to discuss with participants logic and critical thinking in clinical reasoning and decisions, reading, understanding and writing medical articles and theses, improving communication with colleagues and patients, and communicating and positively dealing with physician stress and health[51]. Drs. Dianne Maier (organizer and sponsor from the Alberta Medical Association), Ghazwan Altabbaa ( from the University of Calgary and its Department of Medicine, moderator and initiator of the project), and Milos Jenicek (presenter) participated in their respective roles.

The objective of the encounters was coverage and knowledge of basic rules of informal logic and critical thinking in medical practice and research. In terms of attitudes, participants were led to see this field as a useful, structured and necessary way of understanding medical problems and making rational decisions about them. In terms of skills, participants learned how to critically analyze clinical situations and selected medical information pertaining to them, to apply the critical thinking methodology at least in part to problems of their choice and to evaluate for themselves the correctness and relevance of such an experience. Selected major fallacies in medical reasoning and decision-making were highlighted and corrections proposed.

A seminar form with group discussion on selected major fallacies in reasoning and decision-making were the major teaching methods. PowerPoint© presentations summarizing the message and short practical examples were distributed at each encounter to all. The PowerPoint© presentations were based in part on the spirit and style of vignettes and exercises proposed by us in *A Physician's Self-Paced Guide to Critical Thinking.*[38]

The evaluation was formative. About one third of participants gave the program high marks, one third gave average marks and the rest gave low marks reflecting feelings about evidence-based medicine itself. It was felt that in the future, a workshop of at least one-day would be more appropriate for this topic and the mastery of its components.

Both of these experiences were in line with our expectations of what might be expected from these first initiatives devoted to critical thinking as their main topic (how modern critical thinking methodology in health sciences is structured, relevant, teachable and usable in research and practice) and led us to further review the strengths and some weaknesses in evidence-based medicine whose expanded interface with logic and critical thinking methodology appears increasingly more applicable[43,45,52,53].

### 3. How do we foresee teaching critical thinking in medicine in the future in the light of past and present experiences?

Given the experiences past and present discussed above, we work within a solid framework with critical thinking[5] on one side and its steadily improving teaching and evaluation[6] on the other. Some conceptual and methodological elements for medicine are now also available. Several major challenges are anticipated in the near future with regard to methodology and teaching interface.

### Overcoming terminology and methodology overload, overlaps, and discrepancies

An increasing number of new terms are enriching those already in existence in medicine, epidemiology, biostatistics and EBM. Critical thinking and argumentation vocabulary, newer for all, do not simplify the situation. For example, in the field of evidence-based medicine, there are about thirteen definitions for evidence-based medicine itself, two for evidence-based clinical practice, five for evidence-based healthcare, one for evidence-based practice[54] and at least three for evidence-based public health[55-57]. Within epidemiology and biostatistics, at least five definitions for bias are quoted[58]. Moreover, biases overlap in their meaning with what philosophers would call fallacies. In philosophy, numerous synonyms for a great number of fallacies complicate matters for beginners and classifications abound. As for critical thinking itself, more than twenty definitions were compiled[59-61]. In the theory of the scientific method[62, 63], scholars still disagree about the number and sequence of steps that constitute it, going from four[63] to fifteen[62]. Pragmaticians who are accustomed to straightforward definitions of cancer, obstetrics, cardiology, iron deficiency or myocardial infarction often ignore various different types of definitions known to logicians[64]. It will take some time (and a proper clearinghouse) for this often cacophonic tower of Babel to disappear.

## Improving the interface between knowledge, practice, experience and critical thinking as foundations of medical understanding and decision-making

Teaching critical thinking and critical thinking itself should not be offered as a new graft to be accepted or rejected. Critical thinking is a discipline that must be taught and learnt as anything else. It cannot be acquired simply by osmosis from more experienced medical elders. It should be taught by all and learnt by all. However, some methodologically experienced 'critical thinkers' will appear to convey the fundamentals of critical thinking and argumentation by teaching the teachers. They will join the crowd of basic sciences and clinical specialists, epidemiologists, biostatisticians, sociologists and others as "teaching time mongers" in undergraduate programs.

Perhaps the greatest challenge is bedside instruction and floor clinical teaching where we have two choices: Either 'pimping' or teaching argumentation through the Socratic method. Again, both options should be known to all and training in the latter and its practice will not come by itself either. We cannot count solely on the knowledge of critical thinking acquired in our college years. Often, the only information overloaded physicians remember from their elementary logic classes is that *'all humans are mortal – Socrates is human – Socrates is mortal'*. Even if they are better equipped in logic and critical thinking, we cannot assume that they will automatically be able to translate and apply these critical thinking skills in the context of medicine. Hence, critical thinking should be taught in close relation and application to various steps of clinical and epidemiological reasoning[50, 51] and decision making[65, 66] or to the steps of the scientific method and research methodology from original ideas to final claims in the production of new evidence. This medical practice and research adapted methodology in argumentation and critical thinking in its own curriculum will necessarily deviate from a similar curriculum in critical thinking training at large.

So far, teaching of critical thinking in medicine with varying contents and through various teaching methods is already seen throughout the world and has proven to be progressively useful at the undergraduate level,[67-70] in basic sciences,[71] in teaching residents,[72,40] in family medicine,[73,74] and also in health care management,[75,76] and health promotion.[77]

What will appear, then, as teaching and learning proposals in the reader's future? Here are some guidelines for developing effective classroom and bedside teaching sessions that embed critical thinking in the teaching of the health sciences:

- Try to define as clearly as possible the desirable and necessary attitudes, knowledge and skills needed for a clinical practice grounded in critical thinking.
- Develop common objectives, core content and suitable teaching methodology and evaluation of TCTM that would be usable not only in medicine, but also in other health sciences.
- Define the problem and question (differential diagnosis, toxic effect, treatment, effectiveness in an individual or group) in a manageable form for argumentation.
- Gather the best and unbiased evidence as a base from which critical thinking will be applied.
- Incorporate critically appraised evidence into the building blocks of the argument
- Use argument construction or reconstruction as a means leading to the solution of the problem, both carried out by a Socratic method.
- Do not forget that coupling the best evidence with clinical circumstances and patient preferences and values is also a matter of argumentation and that all three elements (evidence / circumstances / preferences) of clinical decision making are by definition building parts of an argument and argumentation.
- Anticipate, prevent, detect and correct fallacies at any step of the scientific method, patient care, health program, professional and non-professional communication.
- Teach critical thinking in medicine with a focus on understanding and solving health and disease problems.
- Evaluate both the beneficial and problematic effects of your teaching and how they improve the learner's practice and research.

Teaching, learning, practicing and evaluating this type of critical thinking in medicine essentially lie ahead of us. Is there any greater award than our patients and communities benefiting in their health and disease from our will to "make sense" of our endeavors?

What we have seen in this chapter is a long journey already started and to be pursued. Its essence may be symbolically compared to the journey of artists-painters from *pointillism* (at the end of the 19$^{th}$ century) in which a picture was constructed from dots, blending at a distance into recognizable shapes and color tones, to today's single bold strokes of the brush across the whole canvas conveying the essence of the artist's message. Aren't our present experiences in teaching critical thinking in medicine the "dots" that should lead us to some kind of unifying TCTM guidelines ("strokes")?

# Attachment

### Combined Statements of Purpose and Abstracts of recent institutes

1. The APHA institute for public health professionals,[50] a one-day workshop: *Evidence-Based Practice: Logic and Critical Thinking in Public Health*

> The purpose of this workshop is to offer participants a basic overview of the principles and methods of modern informal logic and critical thinking as used and required for effective formulation of public health programs and policies, priority setting, implementation, analysis, and evaluation. Logic and critical thinking is becoming a necessary additional companion to epidemiology, biostatistics and other basic sciences, necessary tools for rational public health. It underlies the whole process of understanding of health problems in the community and making decisions about them. The program will show that any important claim in practice, research, administration or health policy making should be the outcome of use of the best evidence in cogent argumentation accompanied by critical appraisal. The presentation of the activities will be conducted throughout with reference to examples from the public health field. As much as possible, participants will be encouraged to bring their own topics to the program. Selected topics will be used for analysis and improvement by all.

2. Discussion with the academic staff in internal medicine (internists in a teaching position)[51]: *Improving communication with colleagues and patients: it's good for everyone's health, including yours*

> Few things are more frustrating and unproductive than not getting one's message across. Arriving at a mutual understanding of the best evidence, its uses and ensuing recommendations and acceptance of diagnosis, treatment, patient risk assessment and prognosis require structured communication and argumentation. Modern rules of argumentation forwarded by logicians and critical thinking experts for general use also apply to medical practice and research as they already advantageously do in law, business and the military arts. Our discussion will show if and how this domain can be further developed

through our experience. Isn't this, after all, a 'logical' extension of Evidence-Based Medicine?

## 3. Discussion with hospital staff (attending physicians)[51]: *Enhancing the Meaning of our Work: Making the most of our communication with patients and peers at rounds, visits and consults*

Competing alternatives, claims, theories and decisions are ubiquitous in our daily work, so how should we deal with the situation? Empowered with the best evidence, experience and knowledge of specific clinical settings, we need to reach a mutually clear and acceptable understanding of patient problems and our medical decisions, both in line with patient values and preferences. We also need to make good decisions in the end. Modern argumentation at the core of critical thinking as recently developed within informal logic and critical thinking in general is built on a half a dozen or so fundamental considerations. These building blocks must be based not only on valid evidence, but also on their applicable link to our decisions and recommendations to our colleagues and patients. Some frequent fallacies, even if well intentioned, will be pointed out to illustrate challenges in our everyday medical communication.

## 4. Half-day workshop for residents in internal medicine,[51]: Communicate and Positively Tackle Your Stress: Critical thinking methodology in clinical practice and research

Physician self awareness and continuing development of personal communication technique and style is important for individual physician health, collegial and professional relationships and generalizes to improved patient care. Effective clinical decision making in Evidence-Based Medicine requires not only critical appraisal of evidence, but also a mastery of structured ways of reasoning leading to the best possible choices for individual patient or group care (hospital and extramural community). In our seminar, we will outline the differences and complementarity of both concepts. We will see how our knowledge and experience can be used to make the best possible bedside decisions and to effectively share our views with peers.

## References

1. Sumner, W.G. *Folkways. A Study of the Sociological Importance of Usages, Manners, Customs, Mores, and Morals.* Boston, MA: Ginn and Co., 1907.
2. .Dewey J. *How We Think.* Boston, Mass.: D.C. Heath, 1910. (Republished by Mineola, NY: Dover Publications, Inc., 1997.
3, Copi IM. *Informal Logic.* New York, NY: Macmillan, 1986.
4. Ennis RH. *Critical Thinking.* Upper Saddle River, NJ: Prentice Hall, 1996.
5. Facione PA. *Critical Thinking: What It Is and Why It Counts.* 2007 Update. Downloadable at no cost at http://www.insightassessment.com
6. Facione PA. *Critical Thinking: A Statement of Expert Consensus for Purposes of Educational Assessment and Instruction.* Executive Summary. *"The Delphi Report".* 22 pages at

http://www.insightassessment.com/pdf_files/DEXadobe.PDF, retrieved on January 5, 2007.
7. Aristotle. *Prior Analytics.* Translated, with introduction, notes, and commentary, by R Smith. Indianapolis, IN: Hackett Publishing Company, Inc., 1989. (Also, read it on the web, translated by AJ Jenkinson, 29 pages at http://classics.mit.edu/Aristotle/prior.html), retrieved on January 7, 2007.
8. Matilal BK. *Logic, Language, and Reality: An Introduction to Indian Philosophical Studies.* Delhi, India: Motilal Banarsidass, 1985.
9. Toulmin S. *The Uses of Argument.* Cambridge, UK: Cambridge University Press, 1968. (Updated edition, 2003).
10. Toulmin S, Rieke R, & Janik A. *An Introduction to Reasoning.* New York: Macmillan, 1979 (2nd Ed,1984).
11. Mill. J. S. *System of Logic.* Vols 7-8 in: Robson JM, ed. *Collected Works of John Stuart Mill.* Toronto, Ont.: University of Toronto Press, 1963. See also: Mill JS. *A System of Logic. Ratiocinative and Inductive. Being a Connected View of the Principles of Evidence and the Methods of Scientific Investigation.* (1843). Eight Edition (Abridged) with Comments in: *John Stuart Mill's Philosophy of Scientific Method.* Edited with an Introduction by Ernest Nagel. New York: Haffner Publishing Co., 1950.
12. Bernard, C. *Introduction à l'étude de la médicine expérimentale.* Paris: Baillière et fils, 1865. See as *An Introduction to the Study of Experimental Medicine.* New York, NY: Macmillan Publishing Co Inc.: 1927.
13. Hill, A.B. (1953). Observation and experiment. *New England Journal of Medicine* 248,:995-1001. (See also: Hill AB. The environment and disease: Association or causation? (1965). *Proc Royal Society of Medicine,*58, 295-300.
14. Yerushalmy, J. & Palmer, C.E. (1959). On the methodology of investigations of etiological factors in chronic diseases. *Journal of Chronic Disease,* 10, 27-40.
15. Ledley, R.S. & Lusted, L. B. (1959). Reasoning foundations of medical diagnosis; symbolic logic, probability, and value theory aid our understanding of how physicians reason. *Science,*130, :9-21.
16. Feinstein, A. R. *Clinical Judgment.* Baltimore, Md: Williams & Wilkins Co., 1967.
17. MacMahon, B. & Pugh, T.F. Causes of entities of disease. In, D. W. Clark & B. MacMahon. *Preventive Medicine.(*pp. 11-18). Boston: Little, Brown, 1967.
18. MacMahon, B. & Pugh, T.F. *Epidemiology. Principles and Methods.* Boston, MA: Little, Brown & Co., 1970.
19. Surgeon General's Advisory Committee on Smoking and Health. *Smoking and Health.* Washington, DC: US Public Health Service, Publication No 1103, 1969.
20. Susser M. *Causal Thinking in the Health Sciences: Concepts and Strategies of Epidemiology.* New York, NY: Oxford University Press, 1973. (See also: Susser M. What is a cause and how do we know one? A grammar for pragmatic epidemiology. (1991). *American Journal of Epidemiology,*133, 635-48.
21. Buck, C. (1975). Popper's philosophy for epidemiologists. *International Journal of Epidemiol,ogy,* **4,** 159-68. (See also: Buck C., Llopis A, Najera E, Terris M Eds. *The Challenge of Epidemiology: Issues and Selected Readings.* Washington, DC: Pan American Health Organization, 1988.
22. Evans, A.S. (1978). Causation and disease. A chronological journey. *American Journal of Epidemiology,*108, 249-57. (See also: Evans, A.S. *Causation and Disease: A Chronological Journey.* New York, NY: Plenum, 1993.
23. Weed, D.L. (1986). On the logic of causal inference. *American Journal of Epidemiology,* 123, 965-78. (See also: Weed, D.L. (2000). Epidemiologic evidence and causal inference. *Hematology Oncolology Clinics of North America,* 14, 97-807.
24. Greenland S, (Ed.) *Evolution of Epidemiologic Ideas: Annotated Reading on Concepts and Methods.* Chestnut Hill, Mass: Epidemiology Resources Inc., 1987.
25. Rothman, K.J. (Ed.) *Causal Inference.* Chestnut Hill, Mass.: Epidemiology Resources Inc., 1988.
26. Elwood, J.M. *Causal Relationships in Medicine.* Oxford and New York: Oxford University Press, 1988.
27. Jenicek, M. *Foundations of Evidence-Based Medicine.* Boca Raton/London/New York/Washington: The Parthenon Publishing Group/CRC Press, 2003.
28. King, L.S. *Medical Thinking: A Historical Preface.* Princeton, NJ: Princeton University Press, 1962.

29. Murphy, E.A. *The Logic of Medicine.* Baltimore, MD: The Johns Hopkins University Press, 1976. (Second edition, 1997)
30. Pellegrino, E.D. & Thomasma, D.C. *A Philosophical Basis of Medical Practice: Toward a Philosophy and Ethics of the Healing Professions.* New York, NY: Oxford University Press, 1981.
31. Wulff, H.R., Pedersen, S.A., & Rosenberg, R. *Philosophy of Medicine: An Introduction.* Oxford: Blackwell Scientific Publications, 1986.
32. Phillips, C.I., (Ed). *Logic in Medicine.* London, UK: BMJ Publishing Group, 1988. (2nd Ed, 1995).
33. Zadeh LA. Knowledge representation in fuzzy logic. Pp. 1-26 in: Yager RR and LA Zadeh eds. *An Introduction to Fuzzy Logic Applications in Intelligent Systems.* Dordrecht, The Netherlands: Kluwer Academic Publishers, 1992.
34. Sadegh-Zadeh, K. (2000). Fuzzy health, illness and disease. *Journal of Med Phil*, 25, 605-38.
35. Jenicek M. *Epidemiology. The Logic of Modern Medicine.* Montreal: EPIMED International, 1995.
36. Horton R. (1998). The grammar of interpretive medicine. *CMAJ,* 158, 245-9.
37. Jenicek, M. & Hitchcock, D.L. *Evidence-Based Practice. Logic and Critical Thinking in Medicine.* Chicago: American Medical Association/AMA Press, 2005.
38. Jenicek, M. *A Physician's Self-Paced Guide to Critical Thinking.* Chicago: American Medical Association (AMA Press), 2006.
39. Halpern, D.F. & Nummedal, S.G. (Eds). (1995). Special issue: Psychologists Teach Critical Thinking. *Teaching of Psychology,* 22(1): February 1995.
40. Grayson, H. Walker Teaching Resource Center, The University of Tennessee at Chattanooga. *Faculty Development. Critical Thinking.* 8 pages at http://www.utc.edu/Administration/WalkerteachingResourceCenter/FacultyDevelopmen.., retrieved Dec 30, 2006.
41. Brancati, F.L. (1989). The art of pimping. *JAMA,* 262, 89-90.
42. Wear, D., Kokinova, M., Keck-McNumty, C., & Aultman, J. (2005). Pimping: Perspectives of 4th year medical students. *Teach Learn Med,* 17(2), 184-91.
43. West Virginia University Department of Family Medicine – Eastern Division. *Users Guide for OSTE: The Socratic Method and Adult learning In a Cultural Competency Clinical Scenario.* 9 pages at www.hsc.wvu.edu/eastern/pdfs/ResidentCurr/. Retrieved on Jan 4, 2007.
44. Gray, H. *Socratic Discussion. 2004 ASPA Conference Report.* 4 pages at http://www.aspa.asn.au/Confs/Aspa2004/socratic.htm, retrieved on September 22, 2006.
45. Paul R. *A Taxonomy of Socratic Questions.* 2 pages at http://www.wolaver.org/teaching/socratic.htm, retrieved on January 3, 2007.
46. Kee, F. & Bickle, I. (2004). Critical thinking and critical appraisal: the chicken and the egg? *Quarterly Journal of Medicine*, 97, 609-614.
47. Jenicek M. (2006). How to read, understand, and write 'Discussion' sections in medical articles. An exercise in critical thinking. *Medical Science Monitor,* 12(6), SR28-36.
48. Jenicek M. (2006). Towards evidence-based critical thinking medicine? Uses of best evidence in flawless argumentations. *Medical Science Monitor,* 12(8), RA149-153.
49. Critical Thinking Community (/cthink). A Working definition of *critical thinking* by Michael Scriven and Richard Paul. 3 pages at http://lonestar.texas.net/~mseifert/crit2.html, retrieved on June 9, 2005.
50. *Evidence-Based Practice. Logic and Critical Thinking in Public Health. An Interactive Workshop.* APHA – Continuing Education Institutes (CEI), Continuing Education Institute # 1003.0. M Jenicek and DL Hitchcock presenters. The 2005 American Public Health Association (APHA) Annual Meeting *"Evidence-Based Policy and Practice",* Philadelphia, PA, December 10, 2005.
51. Alberta Medical Association, University of Calgary (Department of Medicine), Jenicek M, presenter, Altabbaa G, moderator, Maier D, sponsor. *Calgary Seminar Series on Critical Thinking in Medicine,* Calgary, October 18 and 19, 2006.
52. Jenicek, M. (2006). The hard art of soft science: Evidence-based medicine, reasoned medicine or both? *Journal of Eval Clinical Practice*, 12(4), 410-419.
53. Jenicek, M. Evidence-based medicine: Fifteen years later. Golem the good, the bad, and the ugly in need of a review? *Medical Science Monitor,* 12(11), RA241-251.
54. Anonymous compilation. *Definitions of Evidence-Based Medicine/Healthcare/Practice.* 3 pages retrieved from http://www.shef.ac.uk/scharr/ir/def.html, retrieved on January 7, 2007.

55. Jenicek, M. (1997). Epidemiology, evidence-based medicine, and evidence-based public health. *Journal of Epidemiology,* 7(4), 187-97.
56. Jenicek, M. & Stachenko, S. (2003). Evidence-based public health, community medicine, preventive care. *Medical Science Monitor,* 9(2), BR2 – BR8.
57. Brownson, R.C., Baker, E.A., Leet, T.L., & Gillespie, K.N. *Evidence-Based Public Health.* New York and Oxford: Oxford University Press, 2003.
58. Last, J. M. (Ed). *A Dictionary of Epidemiology.* (4$^{th}$ Ed.). Oxford and New York: Oxford University Press, 2001.
59. Murell, G. & Houlihan, P. Critical Thinking Across the Curriculum. *Definitions of Critical Thinking.* 4 pages at http://planet.tvi.edu/ctac/definect.htm, retrieved on May 29, 2006.
60. Fowler, B. *Critical thinking definitions.* (Longview Community College, Critical Thinking Across the Curriculum Project.) 5 pages at http://mcckc.edu/longview/ctac/definitions.htm, retrieved on December 30, 2006.
61. AUSTHINK$^{TM}$, Critical Thinking on the Web. *Definitions of "Critical Thinking".* 6 pages at http://www.austhink.org/critical/pages/definitions.html, retrived on October 7, 2006.
62. Scientific methods. In, *McGraw-Hill Encyclopedia of Science & Technology, Vol. 16 (SAB-SON).* 9$^{th}$ Ed.(pp. 120-122). New York and Chicago: McGraw-Hill, 2002.
63. Answers.com$^{TM}$.*Scientific Method.* Dictionary. 17 pages at http://www.answers.com/topic/scientific-method, retrieved on December 28, 2006.
64. Meaning and definition. Chapter 2, Pp. 33-60 in: Hughes W, Lavery J. *Critical Thinking. An Introduction to the Basic Skills.* Fourth edition. Peterborough, On and Orchard Park, NY: Broadview Press, 2004.
65. Rudnick A. 2004. An introductory course in philosophy of medicine. *MH Online*, 30, 54-56.
66. Szolovits, P. & Pauker, S. G. Categorical and Probabilistic reasoning in Medicine. 6 pages at http://groups.csail.mit.edu/medg/ftp/psz/Bobrow3.html, retrieved on March 26, 2005.
67. Pitkälä, K., Mäntyranta, Strandberg, T.E., Mäkela, M., Vanhanen, H. & Varonen, H. 2000. Evidence-based medicine – how to teach critical scientific thinking to medical undergraduates. *Medical Teacher,*22(1), 22-26.
68. Maudsley, G. & Strivens, J. (2000). Promoting professional knowledge, experiential learning and critical thinking for medical students. *Medical Education*, 34, 535-544.
69. Louhaia P. (2003). Philosophy for medical students – why, what, and how. *Journal of Medical Ethics: Med Hum,* 29, 87-88.
70. Lieberman, S.A., Trumble, J.M., & Smith, E.R. (2000). The impact of structured student debates on critical thinking and informatics skills of second-year medical students. *Academic Medicine,* 75, S84-S86.
71. Abraham, R.R., Upadhya, S., Torke, A., & Ramnarayan, K. (2004). Clinically oriented physiology teaching: strategy for developing critical-thinking skills in undergraduate medical students. *Adv Physiol Educ,* 28, 102-104. Downloaded from ajpadvan.physiology.org on December 2006.
72. Paukert, J..L. (2000). When residents talk and teachers listen: A communication analysis. *Academic Medicine,* 75**,** S65-S67.
73. Oh, R.C. (2003). The Socratic method in medicine – the labor of delivering medical truths. *Family Medicine,* 37(8), 537-9.
74. General Practice Training Tasmania. *Research & Critical Thinking Module.* GPTT Research & Critical Thinking Module. 21 pages at CHECK
75. Gold J, Holman D, Thorpe R. *The Manager as a Critical Reflective Practitioner: Uncovering arguments at work.* 11 pages at http://www.mngt.waikato.ac.nz/ejrot/cmsconfrence/documents/management%20Education/CRITIC2.pdf, retrieved on December 26, 2005.
76. Open Clinical, Knowledge management for medical care. *Argumentation applied to healthcare applications.* 9 pages at http://www.openclinical.org/argumentation.html, retrieved on September 4, 2006.
77. Fennell R. (2003). Using case studies to promote critical thinking in health promotion. *American Journal of Health Education,* 34(5), 291-3.
78. Veugelers, P.J. & Fitzgerald, A.L. (2005); Effectiveness of school programs in preventing childhood obesity *American Journal of Public Health,* 95, 432-5.

# Reflecting on Practice: A Workshop Exercise

## *Kathleen Chirema*

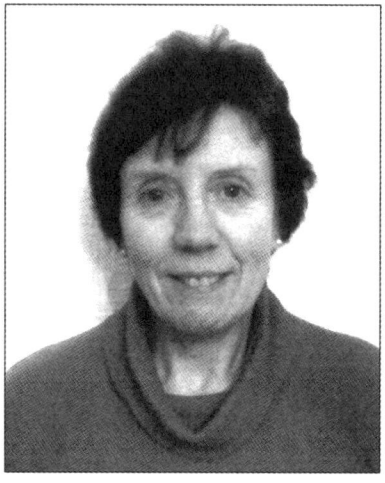

*Dr. Chirema is a Senior Lecturer in the School of Human and Health Sciences Department of Adult and Children's Nursing at the University of Huddersfield, West Yorkshire U.K. She is currently the Course Leader for the BSc [Hons] Professional Studies Degree. This degree is open to a range of Health Care Professionals however, the students are mainly Registered Nurses or Midwives who wish to achieve degree level status following their initial Pre Registration Diploma Programme. Dr. Chirema teaches research methods in a range of modules at Undergraduate and Post Graduate level. She facilitates sessions and workshops on reflective practice in a range of modules. Her research interest focuses on the use of reflective journals to promote reflection on practice and learning from practice experiences in post registration nurses. We are happy to include her pedagogical proposals regarding the importance of reflection in this anthology on teaching.*

**Background on reflection**

Current thinking in nursing advocates the need for nurses to be educated in ways that develop their autonomy, critical thinking skills, sensitivity to others and their open-mindedness (Reid and Ground, 1997). I have found that teaching students reflective thinking strategies is one way of achieving this. Reflection is concentration and careful consideration, and reflective practice is the mindful consideration of one's actions, specifically one's professional actions (Osterman, 1990). The term 'reflective practice' was popularised by Schön (1991). He suggests that coaching can help students learn "the artistry of practice." Schön sees the coaching process as a "ladder of reflection" where students and faculty reflect on their actions, and where a key consideration is balancing challenge and support during reflection. The idea is that one develops the habit of mind of carrying out a focused and critical assessment of one's own practice behaviour as a means of developing one's own craftsmanship.

Reflection is often prompted by a problem, a perceived discrepancy between the real and the ideal, or between what occurred and what was expected. One steps back to examine one's actions as a way of trying to understand the discrepancy. One's task is to reflect on the effectiveness or legitimacy of one's chosen action and to use this new perspective as a means of developing alternate strategies. The entire exercise is an exercise in critical thinking. Johns (2000) suggests that reflection provides nurses with a vehicle through which they can communicate and justify the importance of practice and practice knowledge, thus legitimising the knowledge that derives from the realities of practice. Nursing education has subsequently integrated reflection-on-action into nursing preparation programs and continuing professional development programs for nurses.

The argument that reflection is a critical step in professional development is historically rooted in learning theory. Kolb argued that experience was the basis for learning and that learning could not fully take place without reflection (Kolb, 1984). Kolb described the process of experiential learning as a four stage cycle involving four learning modes: concrete experience, reflective observation, abstract conceptualisation and active experimentation.

Because I think of reflection as a dynamic process, I also like Gibb's reflective framework (1988). This framework offers a series of questions to structure an experience in reflection. Gibb suggests that one should begin by asking, "What happened?" and then proceed with questions that help one to reflect on any important experience. These elements of the reflective process are echoed by Boud, Keogh and Walker (1988): *the returning to experience* (what happened?); *attending to feelings* (how did I feel, why did I act or react this way?); and *re-evaluating experience* (what does it mean?). Figure 1 lists some of the questions proposed by both of these authors for a successful reflection exercise.

1. What happened ? (interpretation)
2. What where you thinking and feeling? (interpretation)
3. What sense can you make of that? (analysis and inference)
4. What else could you have done? (inference and explanation)
5. If the situation arose again, what would you do?

**Figure 1: Questions for Reflection**

## Class session and students

This session would fit well in a staff development programme as an introductory thinking experience within an undergraduate course requiring participants to think critically and reflect on prior learning. I teach the session as part of a module in the School of Human and health Sciences entitled Reflecting on Practice. This honours level workshop permits each student to undertake a different menu of learning and comprises two hours of a 6 hour workshop for students who wish to accredit learning that is not already certificated. The resulting certification can be used to build up credit towards obtaining a degree qualification.

Additionally this module meets the criteria for the Continuing Professional Development (CPD) requirements of the Nursing and Midwifery Council in the United Kingdom and can be taken by Practitioners to undertake additional study around their specialist area and to maintain a professional portfolio to support their practice.

## Goals and objectives for this lesson

One goal for this session is to teach participants to use critical thinking skills to reflect on their learning and to evaluate reflection as a tool for improving their clinical practice. The session takes the form of a independent workshop. The assigned work is aimed at guiding them to think critically about their prior learning and to demonstrate their understanding of some material applicable to clinical practice. Participants carry out an exercise in reflection over a two hour period guided by a packet of assigned materials. Later they undertake a written assignment through which I can assess their ability to use critical thinking skills.

Durghee (1996) argues that through reflection, one is able to analyze clinical situations by breaking them down into significant components and integrating them to achieve patient focused goals. Enthusiastic advocates claim that reflection is generally beneficial to practitioners to optimize their situational awareness, and that it enhances critical thinking, listening and observation skills.

I help the workshop participants to link the reflection lesson to a previous critical incident or significant clinical event. The issues related to a critical incident may have been recorded by the student retrospectively in a reflective journal and subsequently utilized to enhance their learning and to achieve the objectives of this workshop. Participants are encouraged to think critically and utilize the critical thinking skills of analysis, evaluation and self examination.

But no proposed strategy for better thinking should be accepted without careful evaluation of its utility, so one of my goals is to guide the workshop participants to take a fair-minded look at the value of reflection to provide value to their practice. Although reflection has become a major feature of many programmes of adult learning, it is still found to be time consuming and difficult at times, challenging an adults' previous experiences of what learning involves (Dewer, et al., 1994). Perhaps more importantly, others have viewed the reflective process as potentially flawed. Newall (1992), for instance, argues that reflection relies on memory, which may be a major source of practical difficulty because inaccurate recall and anxiety could alter the individual's account of prior events.

## Learning Objectives

By the end of Workshop students should be able to:

- Define reflection as it applies to reflective practice.

- Describe and discuss the critical thinking skills of analysis, evaluation and self examination as they apply to effective reflection on practice.

- Critically evaluate the positive and negative aspects of reflection.

- Analyse and explain how a practitioner would encourage other staff to reflect on practice.

## Material needed for the session

A range of reading materials could be used to prepare workshop participants for this session in reflection on practice. One example would be, "An Introduction to Reflection, the first chapter of *Reflective Practice in Nursing*" by Bulman and Schultz (2004). The material you select should include a section describing and defining reflection. Usually this includes a discussion of types and models of reflection as well as the processes involved. There should also be a discussion of the varying perspectives as to the value of reflection to guide learning about practice in the health sciences.

I forward the assigned readings to the students two weeks before the study session and we use this chapter as a framework for the session. I send them a worksheet to serve as a guide to the areas of reflection to be considered. Journal articles on reflection and reflective practice are available in a folder for participants to use as further reading (Figure 2).

In the workshop I expect all the students to work on the four areas of investigation with a partner. This often increases motivation as they are able to share ideas and discuss options. It also facilitates analysis and evaluation.

---

**Reflection Worksheet**

This exercise is to be completed in small groups or pairs. The exercise focuses on developing your skills in reflection as a clinical reasoning tool. In the course of this exercise you will also be called upon to use your critical thinking skills to analyze the following four areas, interpret the significance of each and explain how it is important to your clinical practice. You and your study partner will have about one hour to complete the questions and tasks on this worksheet. Use the reference file available to you in class to gather evidence together to support your conclusions about the use of critical reflection in practice.

1) Define reflection.

2) Discuss/describe the thinking skills that are required to be able to reflect effectively. You can use everyday language about thinking and decision making in relation to this aspect.

3) What are the positive and negative aspects of reflection?

4) As a Practitioner how would you encourage other staff to reflect?

---

Figure 2: The Worksheet

## What I do before the class begins

It is important to prepare all the materials in advance and I always reread the papers I've asked students to read for the session. I think of the workshop as happening in three stages: 1) giving relevant information, 2) working on the task, and 3) providing feedback to the group. I usually know how many students will attend the session, as well as their area of specialisation. This gives me some insight into their background and their learning needs. I use this knowledge of the group to prepare a range of questions to ask during the feedback stage. I also clearly verbalize my expectations for the Workshop, explaining why each assigned task is being given. This way the students are in no doubt about the significance of the work to be undertaken.

## How do I facilitate this session

I explain that there are four areas of investigation for this worksheet exercise, and ask them to work in pairs. Following my introduction to the content of the workshop I give the students one hour to investigate the four areas under study. I want them to engage the questions energetically and to work in an organised and systematic way to develop the critical thinking dispositions of 'inquisitiveness' and 'systematicity.' In addition to the introductory reading on reflection that they have read before coming to class, I expect students to use other articles on reflective practice that I make available in a resource file in the study area. As they examine these resource materials in light of their experience as practitioners, one person from each pair records key findings and insights on a piece of flip chart paper. Later the large sheets of paper will be fixed to the wall within view of all students, and one student from each pair will provide feedback to the group.

It is my intention to encourage participants to think critically using their skills of analysis, evaluation and explanation, and to exhibit the affective dispositions of self confidence, trust and understanding. The class participants often demonstrate a wide range of ability and are able to work well together by sharing ideas while working in twos. Workshop participants who are new to reflection, especially those who are students early in their studies in the health sciences, may be limited in their ability to carry out the exercise. Some students need quite a lot of support and guidance from the teacher. I work with each of the student groups to monitor their progress and I answer any questions they may have. Just as with any small group exercise, I check at about the half way stage to ask how they are progressing and remind them of the time and the expectations for an oral presentation of their work in the second hour of the workshop.

On completion of the workshop we will have taken time to interpret the meaning of the questions on the Worksheet related to reflection and to discuss the key areas from each group's perspective. I also take time to note the responses and the meaning of each student's contribution as a way of building their self confidence, their trust in their own work and that of their collaborating student. Those who are more experienced with reflection can be expected to carry out this exercise more independently, integrating their knowledge of reflection and its application to practice.

During the second hour of the session I facilitate the feedback from the students. Every student is expected to offer some contribution during this feedback session. Occasionally I add to and support the discussion by my comments and clarifications of areas of difficulty but my primary role is to act as a resource and support the students when they seek clarification in the areas under discussion. As a part of this feedback, I ask the students to talk a bit about their thought processes during the exercise. This request helps to train metacognition and also assists me in making a judgement regarding their critical thinking skills development. Finally, I collate all the comments and let the students have a printed copy of feedback which includes the feedback overall from each of the pairs.

**The Final Work Product**

I often conduct this workshop for students who are authenticating learning experiences that they have completed, so a written component of the lesson is appropriate. There are three main sections: an introduction discussing reflection, and two writing tasks that involve a description of their learning experiences and an analysis and evaluation of a critical incident or significant clinical event.

In the first section I ask the participants to think critically about reflection and to write about their analysis of the relevance of reflective practice for themselves as practitioners and how it may enhance the quality of the care they provide. This portion of the assignment asks that they reference relevant literature in the field. This section is brief, perhaps no more than 250 words.

In the second section the students authenticate twenty hours of learning that has not been previously accredited. They must provide evidence that they have undertaken the learning by including a copy of the related transcript. They must also discuss the nature of the learning activity, giving a well written description of the activity and the outcome of the activity. Again this section can be brief (250 Words).

The third section of this exercise is a piece of academic writing that is an exercise in reflection about a particular clinical episode that they believe provided them significant learning. This episode may be a critical incident or some other significant clinical event. Figure 3 is a suggested format for this part of the written assignment. I expect that students will demonstrate evidence of critical thinking (analysis and evaluation of their current practice) and that they will cite relevant references. I have indicated in brackets the critical thinking skills emphasized when focusing on a critical incident/significant event. This reflection is suggested to be about 1500 words in length.

1) Facts related to the Critical Incident / Significant Event.
- What happened? (Interpretation and Analysis)
- What about it made it "Critical" or "Significant" (Evaluation and Explanation)
- Where and when did it happen? (Description)
- How did it happen? (Analysis and Explanation)

2) Reflect on these associated aspects:
- Your immediate feelings…
- The questions raised by yourself/others…
- What you have learned (Analysis)…
- Your identified additional learning needs (Evaluation)…
- The application of this reflection to your practice…
- How you implemented this new learning into your practice…

**Figure 3: Format for Writing about a Critical Incident / Significant Event**

## Student Response

Students produce the written response to the assignment two months after completion the workshop. The students overall respond well to this type of Workshop. Some do however experience some difficulty in writing reflectively. In evaluating their written response to the introduction and the written analyses of research findings or critical incident, I look for evidence of reflection. I also identify examples of where they have demonstrated the critical thinking skills of analysis and evaluation in all sections of the assignment. Overall the students comment that they appreciate this type of assignment as the experience gained helps them demonstrate the development of both their critical thinking skills and their ability to reflect on learning from experience. Some students, however, find this assignment most challenging – perhaps indicating a need for more practice explaining their thinking processes to others.

## Reference List

Andrews, M. (1996). Using Reflection to develop Clinical Expertise. *British Journal of Nursing* 5(8), 508-513.

Atkins, S. & Murphy, K. (1993). Reflection: Review of Literature *Journal of Advanced Nursing* 18, 1180–1192.

Bolton, G. Reflective Practice, *Writing and Professional Development* London, Sage Publishing, 2005.

Boud, D., Keogh, R. & Walker, D.. *Reflection: Turning Experience into Learning*, London, Keogh Page, 1985.

Boyd, E. M. & Fales, A. W. (1983). Reflective Learning: Key to learning from experience. *Journal of Humanistic Psychology,* 23 (2), 99-117.

Bulman, C. & Schutz, S. *Reflective Practice in Nursing.* 3rd Ed. Blackwell Publishing, 2004.
Burns, S. & Bulman, C.*Reflective Practice in Nursing. Growth of the Reflective Practitioner.* 2nd Ed. Oxford. Blackwell Publishing, 2000.
Chirema, K.D. (2006). The use of reflective journals in the promotion of reflection and learning in post-registration nursing students. *Nurse Education Today,* 27, 192-202.
Clinton, M. (1998). On Reflection Action: Unaddressed issues in refocusing the debate on Reflective Practice. *International Journal of Nursing Practice.* 4, 197 – 202.
Dewer, K. Hill, Y.& MacGregor, J. (1994). Continuing education for nurses, orientating practitioners towards learning. *Adult Learning.* 5 (10), 253-254.
Durgahee,T. (1996). Promoting reflection in Post–Graduate Nursing: A theoretical Model. *Nurse Education Today*, 18, 158-164.
Fowler, J. & Chevannes, M. (1998). Evaluating the efficacy of reflective practice within the context of clinical supervision. *Journal of Advanced Nursing,* 27, 379 – 382.
Freshwater, D. *Therapeutic Nursing – Improving Patient Care Through Self-Awareness and Reflection.* London, U.K.: Sage Publishing, 2002.
Gibb, G. *Learning by Doing: A Guide to Teaching and Learning Methods* Oxford Polytechnic, Oxford Press, 1988
James, C.R. & Clarke, B.A. 1994. Reflective practice in nursing: Issues and implications for nurse education. *Nurse Education Today,* 14, 82-90.
Jasper, M. (2001). The role of the nurse manager in ensuring competence – the use of portfolios and reflective writing. *Journal of Nursing Management*, 9, 249-251.
Johns, C. (1999) Reflection as empowerment? *Nursing Inquiry,* 6, 241 – 249.
Johns, C. *Becoming a Reflective Practitioner. A Reflective and Holistic Approach to Clinical Nursing, Practice Development and Clinical Supervision.* Oxford. Blackwell Science, 2000.
Johns, C. *Guided Reflection Advancing Practice.* Oxford. Blackwell Science, 2002.
Kolb, D. *Experimental Learning: Experience as a source of Learning.* London: Prentice Hall, 1984.*The PREP Handbook.* Nursing and Midwifery Council London: 2002
Newall, R. (1992). Anxiety, accuracy and reflection; the limits of professional development. *Journal of Advanced Nursing,* 17,1326 -1333.
Osterman, K.E. (1990) Reflective Practice - A new agenda for education. . *Education and Urban Society*, 22(2), 133-152.
Palmer, A., Burns, S., Bulman, C. *Reflective Practice in Nursing: The growth of the Professional Practitioner.* Oxford: Blackwell Scientific, 1994.
Perry, M.A. (2003) Reflections on Intuitions and Expertise. *Journal of Advanced Nursing*, 9(1), 137 – 145.
Reid, J.& Ground, I. *Philosophy in Nursing.* London . Arnold Publishing, 1997
Rolfe, G., Freshwater, D. & Jasper, M. *Critical Reflection for Nursing and the Helping Professions: A User's Guide.* Hampshire. Palgrave Publishing, 2001
Rolfe, G. (2002) Reflective Practice: Where now? *Nurse Education in Practice,* 2, 21 – 29.
Schön, D. *The Reflective Practitioner (2nd Ed.)*, San Francisco. Jossey Bass, 1991.
Smith, A. (1998). Learning about reflection. *Journal of Advanced Nursing.*28(4), 891 – 898.
Taylor, B.J. *Reflective Practice: A Guide for Nurses and Midwives).* Open University Press, 2006
Taylor, C. (2003). Narrating practice: Reflective accounts and the textual construction of reality. *Journal of Advanced Nursing.* 42(3), 244 – 251.
Teekman, B. (2000). Exploring Reflective Thinking in Nursing Practice. *Journal of Advanced Nursing.* 31(5), 1125 – 1135.
White, S., Fooks, J., & Gardener, F. *Critical Reflection in Health and Social Care.*Open University Press, 2006

# Evaluating a Nutritional Supplement with SOAP Notes to Develop CT Skills

## Greg A. Brown

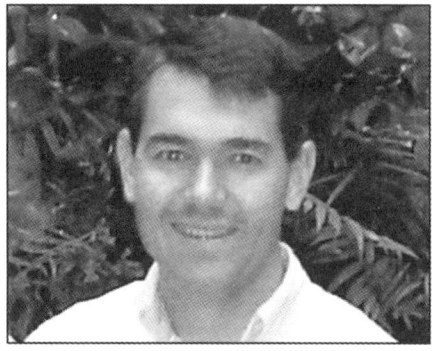

*Dr. Greg. Brown is an Associate professor of Exercise Science at the University of Nebraska at Kearney, College of Education, Dept. of Health, Physical Education, Recreation, and Leisure Studies (HPERLS). He is a member of the American College of Sports Medicine, the American Physiological Society, the National Strength and Conditioning Association, and Sigma Xi the Scientific Research Society. Dr. Brown has published 12 peer reviewed papers evaluating the safety and efficacy of nutritional supplements, so it is no surprise that this lesson has the major focus of nurturing the high level critical thinking skill of evaluation. Mastery of this skill is a central component of achieving competence in clinical reasoning.*

*Like many of the other chapters of this book you will see that Dr. Greg Brown stages this exercise, first talking with students about the strategy that will be used (a SOAP note) to analyze the class material(advertisements about nutritional supplements). Then, once the strategy is understood, it is practiced, evaluated and then practiced again. Most importantly there is a debriefing of the process that includes a specific discussion about how students thought through the exercise and an expectation that they will be able to articulate the reasons behind their judgments. We really like this staged approach that guides students through an analysis and evaluation process on a content area where they are sure to have interest. Dr. Brown's style of requiring his students to provide an explanation of their work is a model for teaching for thinking.*

## Background

The use of nutritional supplements to enhance health or physical appearance is widespread (Kibble, Hansen, & Nelson, 2006; Mason, Giza, Clayton, *et. al.*, 2001; Allen, Thomson, Emmerton *et. al.*, 2000). Frequently, the advertisements for nutritional supplements contain claims and testimonials that sound extremely attractive to consumers; yet these claims may or may not be supported by scientific evidence (Brown, Vukovich, & King, 2006; Froiland, Koszewski, Hingst, *et. al*., 2004; Kamber, Baume, Saugy, *et. al*., 2001). Because of confusion regarding the advertised claims for nutritional supplements, consumers frequently ask health care professionals about the safety and effectiveness of nutritional supplements (Brown, *et. al.,* 2006; Froiland, *et. al*., 2004). Therefore it is important for students in health related majors, such as physical education, health education, nutrition, exercise science, and the medical fields to know how to analyze and compare the advertised claims with the available objective scientific facts about nutritional supplements. The session asks students to use SOAP notes to evaluate a nutritional supplement.

***Class session and students:*** This paper describes an assignment that has been used successfully in an undergraduate class titled "Nutrition for Health and Sport" to help students develop critical thinking skills by using SOAP notes to evaluate a nutritional supplement. Prior to taking this class, students have taken introductory nutrition, anatomy & physiology and exercise physiology, as well as other classes in chemistry, physics, and biology, and most students are in their 6th – 8th semester (late junior to senior years) in college. At this point they have mastered an adequate amount of theoretical and practical content knowledge in nutrition that can be used to address the analysis and evaluation of the advertisement and I am calling on them to use this content knowledge to inform the critical thinking learning activity.

**Learning Objectives for the Project**

1) At the completion of this course, students will be able to interpret advertised claims about a specific nutritional supplement, research these claims in the scientific literature, and analyze the benefits and harms associated with the supplement.

2) Students will develop a plan for assessing the efficacy and safety of a nutritional supplement using the SOAP note strategy and practice this strategy by evaluating one nutritional supplement in depth.

3) Students will demonstrate the critical thinking skills of *interpretation* (of the claims about the supplement), *inference* (about potential risks and benefits), *analysis* (of the information provided by the supplement), and an *evaluation* based on research of why they see the supplement as safe, beneficial, or unsafe, non-beneficial.

As indicated above, although the scientific support for their claimed benefits may be sparse, the use of nutritional supplements to enhance health, physical appearance and athletic performance is widespread. One age old and commonly used tool in the medical field for the comparison of the advertised claims with objective scientific facts for a product is SOAP notes (Kibble, *et. al.*, 2006). The SOAP in SOAP notes stands for **S**ubjective **O**bjective **A**ssessment **P**lan (Sleszynski, Glonek & Kuchera, 1999). In this assignment the students will use SOAP notes to evaluate a dietary supplement that is claimed to enhance health or exercise performance. By using SOAP notes as a strategy to guide their thinking when evaluating a nutritional product, a health professional can compare advertised claims with scientific facts about the product. The evaluation will be helpful to both the student themselves and consumers who they may later counsel.

*Important:* It is not suggested or required that the students purchase the supplement that they are analyzing. And it is stressed that I am not advocating their personal use of any of the supplements that are being evaluated by the class. Students often look to me to validate their assessments of particular products, and this is a teaching moment for critical thinking. If I simply answer 'yes' that's right or 'no' that's wrong, I risk communicating that their own evaluation is less adequate. For this to be a critical thinking exercise, I need to be sure that the emphasis is not on me as expert, but on them as evaluator. Rather then simply questioning me, they need to draw their own inferences about the product and seek out their own evidence for the evaluative judgment they are asked to make.

**General Overview of the Project**

Just to be sure everyone in the class is familiar with the SOAP note process, I begin the classroom discussion with a description of a SOAP note and how one thinks through the process of writing one. I give the students an example of a well written SOAP note by developing one in class using PowerPoint.

As a part of this lesson I ask students to evaluate one nutritional supplement that is of interest to them and to consider its value for their own personal use. I give them guidelines for this task (SOAP Notes OVERVIEW). They are encouraged to think in terms of their own lives and personal characteristics (age, gender, lifestyle, fitness, disease risk or symptoms, body composition, etc.). This assures that the case history of the client that they are analyzing is familiar to the student and can easily be incorporated into the SOAP notes process. Otherwise those students who were not adept at taking case histories would be overly challenged by the exercise. Providing a target audience for the students helps them tailor the tone of their writing.

This project is spread across a semester with the students completing the assignment in stages. The students use content knowledge that they are mastering in other parts of the course or in other parts of their programs. There are four stages to this exercise, each stage completed and turned in following a class discussion of the new part of the exercise, highlighting the goals and concepts included in the stage. Students have several weeks to research and prepare each of the stages.

After the students have submitted each stage, it is reviewed, graded, and returned to the student with comments to help improve the complete SOAP note that will be submitted at the end of the semester. The timeline indicated below is based on a 16 week semester.

The students are given two weeks to complete stage 1, which is simply some personal information and the selection of a supplement to evaluate. Then they have three weeks to complete stage 2, which involves finding advertisements and information about the supplement from popular media. Stage 3 is one of the more challenging parts of the project, because it requires the students to find peer reviewed research data regarding their supplement (four weeks). Stage 4 requires the students to complete the exercise by comparing and evaluating the popular media information and advertisements for the supplement against the scientific data using the resources they have gathered (two weeks). Then a complete SOAP Note document on their supplement, with revision based upon instructor comments, is submitted in the last week of the semester.

Students are given the following SOAP Notes overview in the syllabus on the first day of class and Tables 1-4 are provided to the students as a separate detailed assignment description with the due dates for each stage listed. The students are then given more specific details and an example each time we begin a new stage of the exercise. Each state must be completed before we can optimally begin the next component of the exercise, so I stress the importance of working through the exercise completing each stage on time.

**SOAP Notes Stage 1: Personal Information**

In class, we discuss why people use and buy supplements. In general, supplements are used to improve the health of the person taking the supplement (Allen, *et. al.*, 2000; Kibble, *et. al.*, 2006). This often leads to an interesting discussion with students who have used supplements and have or have not noticed effects (either positive or negative) associated with their supplement use. It is then explained to the students that they need to evaluate their health and lifestyle in order to identify a reason they may want to try and use a nutritional supplement much like a consumer would before choosing a supplement. So, for the next two weeks, students are instructed to evaluate their health, fitness, and lifestyle as completely and possible in order to identify something that they may wish to enhance through supplement use, and select an appropriate supplement. The assignment for evaluating the personal health includes completing the information in Table 1.

| Table 1 of your SOAP Notes: Personal Information |
|---|
| Provide your demographic and health status information and then answer all the remaining questions as completely as possible. <br><br> 1. Student Name <br> 2. Gender <br> 3. Age <br> 4. Body Height <br> 5. Body Mass <br> 6. What is your Body Mass Index or percent body fat? How does your body composition rate based on established norms? <br> 7. What is your $VO_2max$? <br> 8. How does your aerobic fitness rate based on established norms? <br> 9. What is your strength to body mass ratio for bench press and leg press? <br> 10. How does your muscular fitness rate based on established norms? <br> 11. How often do you exercise and what type of exercise do you do? <br> 12. Do you have any known illnesses or allergies that may influence the desirability or safety of using a nutritional supplement? <br> 13. Are there any other lifestyle or health factors that may influence your need for a supplement? <br> 14. What is the name for the supplement you have chosen to evaluate? <br> 15. What is the main (or active) Ingredient? <br> 16. Are the any other ingredients? If so, what are they? <br> 17. Why did you select this supplement, and how might it enhance your health? |

## SOAP Notes Stage 2: Subjective Information

Each student identifies an advertisement for the supplement they plan to review. I help them locate Internet sites making claims about or advertizing nutritional supplements. Another good source of this information is the *Sports Supplement Review* (Phillips, 1997). It is important, of course, that the example I use as my own in class is not one that any of the other students will be using for their project. I want them to use the thinking strategies that I demonstrate on their new problem case.

Each student presents their analysis of their advertisement, describing the health claims being made about the supplement. Then, as a class, we begin to evaluate these claims ('well grounded' or 'too good to be true'). Through this discussion students see that nutritional supplements are frequently advertised with testimonials as evidence of safety and efficacy, but that these testimonials are not always well supported with sound data or science. They also observe that many supplements are advertised with very technical sounding descriptions that are intended to impress the average consumer with scientific jargon and terminology. Over the next three weeks I challenge them to explore, analyze, and assess for themselves all of the claims contained in the advertisement. They begin with a Subjective assessment (Table 2), responding in a narrative style, or short answer responses by questions number. Personally, I like students to write most of the SOAP note in a narrative style.

| Table 2 of your SOAP Notes: Subjective Information |
|---|
| Assess the claims or advertisements about the supplement on the basis of the popular literature and the internet (not the literature from your own reading of scientific journals at this point). You can search aggressively in all other published materials for this information. Your assessment must include references to at least one website that is directly selling the supplement, one "informational" website that is not directly selling the product, one resource from a non-scientific journal (e.g. *Runners World*, *Muscle and Fitness*, *Reader's Digest,* etc) and one news article from a source such as *CNN*, *Time*, *Newsweek*, etc (this may be an internet source for news such as Yahoo! news). |

Answer all questions as completely as possible.

1. What sources of information do you have about the supplement?
2. Are they primarily companies selling the supplement, or are these sources just providing information about the supplement?
3. Is the supplement a single ingredient supplement or does it have many ingredients? What are they?
4. What is the function of each ingredient?
5. What claims are being made for the supplement?
6. Is this supplement "specially formulated" in any way that is purported to enhance efficacy?
7. Who are the target consumers for the supplement? Who should or should not use the supplement?
8. What have you been told about the supplement by friends or sales people?
9. Who produces the supplement? What is the producer's reputation (if known)?

## SOAP Notes Stage 3: Objective Information

I've learned that I need to help students think about how they will objectively evaluate their chosen nutritional supplement. The objective assessment draws upon their knowledge of anatomy, physiology, and nutrition, as well as other sources of information that were not used in the Subjective assessment. I find it helps the students if we practice this part of the assignment together using an example such as androstenedione, which was claimed to increase testosterone and strength without any negative side effects. In fact, the research indicates that these claims are almost completely without scientific merit (Brown, *et. al.*, 2006: King, Sharp, Vukovich, *et. al.*, 1999). The purpose of this discussion is not to convince students that nutritional supplements are ineffective or unsafe, but more to educate the students that distortions are common in the advertisements. Frequently the claims made for nutritional supplements are either exaggerations of what has been found through research, or the claims only mention the positive findings from research and either downplay or ignore the negative findings.

Some key content for this portion of the lesson is the legal definition of a nutritional supplement as defined by the Dietary Supplement Health and Education Act (DSHEA) of 1994 (FDA, US. Gov. 1995). Under DSHEA, as nutritional supplement is defined as

- a product (other than tobacco) that is intended to supplement the diet that bears or contains one or more of the following dietary ingredients: a vitamin, a mineral, an herb or other

- botanical, an amino acid, a dietary substance for use by man to supplement the diet by increasing the total daily intake, or a concentrate, metabolite, constituent, extract, or combinations of these ingredients.
- is intended for ingestion in pill, capsule, tablet, or liquid form.
- is not represented for use as a conventional food or as the sole item of a meal or diet.
- is labeled as a "dietary supplement."
- includes products such as an approved new drug, certified antibiotic, or licensed biologic that was marketed as a dietary supplement or food before approval, certification, or license (unless the Secretary of Health and Human Services waives this provision).

Furthermore, claims may not be made about the use of a dietary supplement to diagnose, prevent, mitigate, treat, or cure a specific disease. Knowing this, the students can now also evaluate whether the supplement that they are reviewing is in compliance with this standard.

Although students should know how to find and evaluate scientific literature at this point in their academic career, I also find it useful to demonstrate how to search a scientific database, such as PubMed, for scientific findings about a given supplement and also how to find the literature in the university library. An in class discussion of a primary research article about a nutritional supplement can also be useful to help solidify the students understanding of how to read primary research literature. It is also useful to discuss with students some basic of research design, such as double blind and placebo control, and why these concepts are so important when testing a product for safety and efficacy.

This part of the project is more difficult for many students, as they may have difficulty finding or reading the scientific literature relevant to their supplement. During this stage is when students express the most frustration as they frequently discover that the scientific literature regarding their supplement is not as clear or prevalent as would appear from the subjective information. I have found that four weeks for this stage allows the students enough time to do a literature search, retrieve their sources, and synthesize answers to the questions. It is also important to have a mid-stage progress report, a consultation with the instructor, or at least an in-class discussion about how the students are progressing.

**Table 3 of your SOAP Notes: An Objective evaluation of the supplement**

**Objective:** Assess the safety and efficacy claims about the nutritional supplement by consulting the scientific literature yourself. You must include references to at least 5 peer reviewed research articles. These cannot be editorials or opinion pieces. Use only research studies about the supplement in which variables are measured and an hypothesis is tested, and accepted or rejected. Ideally the studies should be testing the claims made by the advertisements. You are also encouraged to consult DSHEA guidelines and NIH Office of Dietary Supplement fact sheets, but these do not count towards the required 5 peer-reviewed articles.

Answer all of these questions as completely as possible using your scientific sources. Your answers should not just be 'yes' or 'no' responses. You will need to <u>explain why</u> and reference your scientific source.

1. Are the supplement claims in accordance with DSHEA guidelines for what a supplement can or cannot claim to do or be?
2. Is the supplement safe?
3. What are the possible negative side effects to using the supplement?
4. What is known about the efficacy of the supplement? (e.g. does the supplement do what is claimed, if so, how well?)
5. Does the preparation method affect potency or safety?
6. What does the active ingredient do?
7. What is known about each ingredient (if there are multiple ingredients)?
8. Are there any known synergistic or antagonistic effects of the ingredients?
9. What is the recommended dose? Is there a safe, or tolerable upper limit for the ingredients in the supplement?
10. What is the medical or biological need for the supplement?
11. Are there contraindications to using the supplement?
12. How might your health or fitness affect the effectiveness and safety of the supplement?
13. What is the likelihood of an adverse reaction to the supplement?

## SOAP Notes Stage 4: Assessment and Plan

The final stage for the SOAP notes assignment is where the students focus their critical thinking skills on a comparison of the advertised claims with the research findings. This is the place where they are asked to examine all of the information that they have found about the supplement and make a judgment about whether the supplement in question is safe and, if so, whether it will help them realize their health goals. The students are also asked to develop a plan for monitoring the safe use of the supplement if it was to be adopted for use for themselves or others. They need to explain how they would monitor safety and efficacy. The questions in Table 4 help guide the students through this stage.

A key concept in this stage is to impress students is that they must support their judgment with an evidence base. It will not be enough to simply state "I think this supplement..." without supporting such a statement with findings from the scientific literature. I also find that some students even need to be given a sentence format to help them think clearly about how they will present the report. I suggest that they could use a statement such as "Supplement X is advertised to do Y and Z. However, so and so (cite a reference) observed that neither of these occurred when subjects were administered the supplement in a dose of XX. Instead, W occurred in the subjects." If the time in the course allows, I ask each student to make an in-class presentation on their supplement. This presentation can be very brief, including a discussion of what the supplement was advertised to do, what the research indicates about the safety and efficacy of the supplement, and their assessment and plan for using the supplement (or warning against the supplement). Preparation for a short oral presentation is another way to practice critical thinking skills because students will need to compose a clear description of the supplement and its proposed effects and also compose their arguments about risks and benefits about the supplement and defend their plan for monitoring its use.

## Assessment

Student responses for any of these Stages could serve as classroom level assessment data. They can be examined later by me or anyone for evidence of demonstrated critical thinking skills (analysis, inference, evaluation). Asking for a thorough response to many questions that require critical thinking provides ample evidence of the students' critical thinking skills for this type of analysis.

## Table 4 of your SOAP Notes:
## An Assessment of the Supplement and a Plan for Safe Use

**Assessment:** This is the most important part of the project. Compare the advertised claims with the research. Determine if the supplement is safe and effective or not, and discuss why you are making this judgment. Notice that these are not the same things, so you will need to provide BOTH a discussion of safety and a discussion of efficacy.

Answer all of these questions as completely as possible
1. Are the advertised claims in agreement with the scientific knowledge regarding the supplement? Why or why not?
2. What are the benefits associated with taking the supplement?
3. What are the risks associated with taking the supplement?
4. What evidence is there to support the use of this supplement? (In essence, summarize the claims relative the to scientific facts)
5. Should this supplement be eliminated from consideration? Why or why not? (be specific)

**Plan:** This is also an important consideration. Using your knowledge of health science develop a plan for monitoring the safety and efficacy of the supplement for those who elect to use this supplement. Make the plan as if you would use the supplement. That is, use your own demographic and health status data provided in Stage 1 to make this monitoring plan:

Answer all of these questions as completely as possible

1. How will potential side effects be monitored? (What exactly will you measure and when?)
2. How will side effects be reported?
3. What dose will be administered? Why?
4. How long will the supplement be used? Why?
5. How will effectiveness be monitored? (What exactly will you measure and why?)
6. When and how will the supplement be discontinued if effectiveness is not demonstrated or safety becomes an issue? (Describe in detail)

Quite a number of critical thinking dispositions are also called into play in this exercise (Facione & Facione, 1996). Most assignments that ask students to research the popular and scientific literature are aimed at increasing their inquisitiveness. The SOAP is a systematic approach to the analysis of the supplement, and so the exercise practices the students in systematicity. Finally, the structure of this exercise asks students to suspend their judgment about the supplement until they have searched several sources of information. Even though they might prematurely judge the supplement either safe and efficacious or the opposite, the SOAP note format encourages a reconsideration and demands that students explain why they judge the supplement as safe/unsafe or efficacious/not efficacious. I'm challenging them to develop the cognitive maturity needed to reconsider in the face of new evidence. And, of course, courageously seeking the best possible knowledge regarding the supplement means that they are developing and reinforcing the disposition of truth-seeking.

Many other outcomes are also achieved. After using the SOAP notes technique, in addition to increasing their knowledge of the safety and efficacy for a specific nutritional supplement, the students will have developed their skills in reading scientific literature and in critically evaluating a nutritional product using their health science knowledge.

## Student Feedback

I have received many favorable comments about this assignment from my students. Many students say that they did not realize how scarce the research is on many products sold as nutritional supplements. Others say that they assumed that nutritional supplements were subject to the same testing and research as prescription medications, but they have learned through this assignment that supplements are instead regulated like food products with no requirement for pre-marketing research. I always like to conclude this assignment by telling the students that nutritional supplements may or may not enhance health. Some supplements have quite solid evidence supporting their advertised claims, some supplements have had their claims refuted by solid science and in many cases the research is insufficient to either accept or reject the advertised claims. Overall, the best advice one can take when considering nutritional supplements is "Caveat Emptor" (let the buyer beware).

## References

Allen, T., Thomson, W.M., Emmerton, L.M. & Poulton, R. (2000). Nutritional supplement use among 26-year-olds. *New Zealand Medical Journal*, 113, 274-277.

Brown, G.A., Vukovich, M. & King, D.S. (2006). Testosterone prohormone supplements. *Medical Sciences Sports Exercisec,* 38, 1451-1461.

Froiland, K., Koszewski, W., Hingst, J. & Kopecky, L. (2004). Nutritional supplement use among college athletes and their sources of information. *International Journal of Sports Nutrition and Exercise Metabolism,* 14, 104-120.

Kamber M, Baume N, Saugy M and Rivier L. Nutritional supplements as a source for positive doping cases? *Int J Sport Nutr Exerc Metab* , Vol. 11: 258-263, 2001.

Kibble, J., Hansen, P.A. & Nelson, L. (2006). Use of modified SOAP notes and peer-led small-group discussion in a Medical Physiology course: addressing the hidden curriculum. *Advanced Physiological Education*, 30, 230-236.

King, D.S., Sharp, R.L., Vukovich ,M.D., Brown, G.A., Reifenrath, T.A., Uhl, N.L. & Parsons, K. A. (1999). Effect of oral androstenedione on serum testosterone and adaptations to resistance training in young men: a randomized controlled trial. *JAMA,* 281, 2020-2028.

Mason, M.A., Gizam M., Clayton, L., Lonning, J. & Wilkerson, R.D. (2001). Use of nutritional supplements by high school football and volleyball players. Iowa *Orthopedics Journal,* 21, 43-48.

Phillips B. *Sports Supplement Review* (3rd ed). Mile High Publishing, Golden CO 1997.

Sleszynski, S.L., Glonek, T. & Kuchera, W.A. (1999). Standardized medical record: a new outpatient osteopathic SOAP note form: validation of a standardized office form against physician's progress notes. *Journal of the American Osteopathic Assoc,* 99, 516-529.

U. S. Food and Drug Administration, Center for Food Safety and Applied Nutrition, Dietary Supplement Health and Education Act of 1994, December 1, 1995 http://www.cfsan.fda.gov/~dms/dietsupp.html, accessed January 22, 2007.

## Some Interesting Links about Supplements

NIH ODS Dietary Supplement Fact Sheets
   http://dietary-supplements.info.nih.gov/Health_Information/Information_About_Individual_Dietary_Supplements.aspx

Are Herbal Supplements Hurting You? New Book Says It's A Buyers-Beware Market For Herbal Remedies CBS Evening News, January 15, 2007
   http://www.cbsnews.com/stories/2007/01/15/eveningnews/main2359540.shtml?source+RSSattr=Health_2359540

How Should FDA Regulate Diet Supplements? Dietary Supplement Health And Education Act Regulates Supplements As Foods, Not Drugs CBS Evening News, January 16, 2007
   http://www.cbsnews.com/stories/2007/01/16/eveningnews/main2364595.shtml

# From "What" to "Why" – Reflective Storytelling as Context for Critical Thinking

## *Susan Gross Forneris & Susan Ellen Campbell*

*Drs. Susan Gross Forneris and Susan Ellen Campbell are both faculty in the Department of Nursing at the College of St. Catherine in St. Paul Minnesota, USA.*

*Dr.Gross Forneris' [right] has been examining the relationship between context-based analysis of clinical cases and improved critical thinking in practice. Her clinical expertise is in rehabilitation, case management and leadership. When she trains clinical reasoning in the classroom and clinic, she always focuses on* 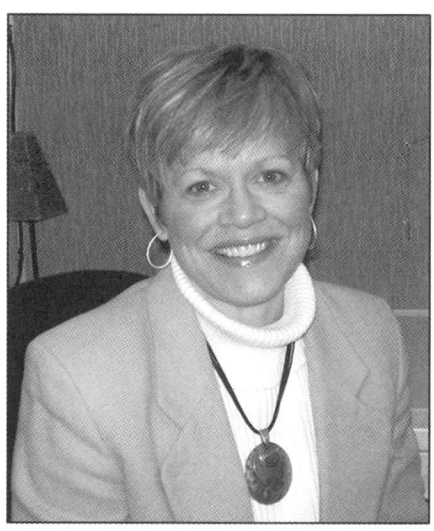 *developing skill in meta-cognition. Thinking about and evaluating one's thinking guards patients from error and protects clinicians in the workplace.*

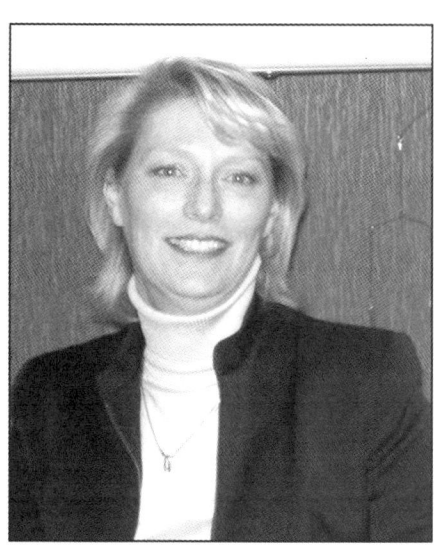

*Professor Susan Ellen (Suellen) [left]Campbell's clinical expertise is medical-surgical nursing. She coordinates post baccalaureate education at the College of St. Catherine. Together, these colleagues use what they term a "thinking nursing" approach based on the theoretical framework proposed by Carper (1978) in her papers on patterns of knowing. Their class exercises strive to include the practice of critical thinking skills to enhance connections between classroom learning and practice.*

**Class session and students:**

Drawing from the nursing education literature on narrative pedagogy (Diekelmann, Ironside & Harlow, 2003; Ironside, 2003) and critical dialogue (Brookfield, 1990, 1995, 2000; Myrick & Yonge, 2004; Myrick, 2002), this class session is part of an introductory baccalaureate nursing assessment course where students are beginning to learn how to assess a clinical case. In this course, stories are integrated into the teaching approach in an effort to begin developing a foundation for students to think within the context of nursing practice. Because we believe that this pedagogical approach is very effective for building critical thinking skills, we introduce this story approach early in the course. The class session we outline here would fit well in any clinical course with health science students involved in beginning clinical experiences.

Creating context assists students' abilities to share their thoughts and feelings about clinical practice experiences and to reflect and make meaningful learning connections. We want them to practice using critical thinking in the context of these stories and make meaningful learning connections. We believe that their successful learning will motivate them to transfer these cognitive behaviors to actual practice. These exercises will facilitate their development to *critically think in practice.*

**The goal of the class session**

Our goal in this course is to facilitate students' ability to be critically reflective and connect the abstract ideas of nursing theory and the unique context of practice. The use of personal stories as a method to enhance students' ability to be critically reflective is derived from the philosophical and theoretical notions of narrative or story. Some of the classic work on narratives was done by Labov (1962). He demonstrated how stories were often told for the purpose of communicating about important dilemmas and problem situations. As a result of telling the story, the storyteller's perspective on a key dilemma and how the storyteller views the resolution of the problem situation is readily apparent. In this case, everything that the storyteller includes in the story provides insight into what the storyteller wants to communicate about the actual experience being captured in the story (Labov, 1962; Reismann, 1993).

We want students to use these aspects of storytelling to better understand their experiences and actions therefore through the use of story, students engage in an active learning process whereby they actively read and reflect on their stories. At the same time the professor is offered a window into the student's understanding of the clinical incident. Through reflection, we focus on the context of the story and, through the use of guiding questions, students begin to understand any implicit meanings. This helps then to intentionally connect their classroom learning with real-life practice. Stories are shared between students in a small seminar class. Our role as faculty is to guide a critically reflective dialogue within the small student discussion group. Stories provide the mechanism for understanding as they can be reflected on, reanalyzed and understood.

In addition to guiding students to use their critical thinking skills in a clinical story context, we also want them to begin to understand something about their thinking process. So we talk with them a bit about critical thinking and problem-solving, and help them make connections between these terms. In this way they begin to more closely focus on their own thinking processes. Our learning objective reflects both of these considerations.

## Learning objectives

Following presentation, discussion and assigned learning activities, the students will be able to:

1. Use elements of story telling to help them analyze and learn from their clinical practice experiences.
2. Improve critical thinking skills (analysis, inference, explanation and evaluate) through stories that they tell about their clinical practice experiences.
3. Analyze and discuss the knowledge that they have gained from actual clinical experiences
4. Discuss the characteristics, skills, and attitudes of the critical thinker, and relationship between the concepts: nursing process, critical thinking, problem-solving and decision-making.

## Students' preparation for this reflective seminar

This exercise has as its aim the integration of knowledge gained in the classroom, the practice of critical thinking skills and the development of skill in clinical reasoning. Initially the students use prepared cases to achieve these learning outcomes. As the course moves along and as students have more opportunity for clinical work, we ask students to journal about an important clinical experience and to submit their stories prior to the seminar day. Figure 1 below is a sample of the assignment guideline that we give to students to help them select, write about, and submit a clinical story. Following the reflective seminar, students then create a written reflection about the learning connections and new insights into their story as a result of sharing and discussing their story with peers and the instructor.

> **Guidelines for Storytelling as Reflective Journaling**
>
> 1. Recall a clinical experience that resulted in a feeling of accomplishment, satisfaction, and/or resulted in feelings of discouragement or frustration. Write about this experience in the form of a story with a beginning, middle and end. To help you provide context for your story, think about the questions "Who?" "What?" "When?" and "Where?" as you write the story.
>
> 2. Following your post-clinical seminar, critically reflect on your story and the discussion about your story with your seminar group. Prepare a written reflection of your clinical story per the guidelines below:
>
> - Why did you pick your story?
> - Discuss the learning connections you made that helped bring what you read and discussed in the classroom more practical and real in the clinical setting.
> - How do you think this story will impact your nursing practice?

**Figure 1: An example of the assignment prompt we give students for this session**

### Our preparation before class for this assignment

In the early weeks of the course, students have had very few clinical experiences prior to and in the first two months of the course. Through student participation in the critical reflection seminar at the end of the semester, we help students to make connections between what they learned early in the course through the use of case studies in the classroom and lab, to what they experienced during their clinical experiences.

We review the stories that the students have submitted for the reflective seminar, and prepare for the guided reflective dialogue that will occur in the seminar by analyzing the stories for their possible meanings. Each instructor works individually with approximately 24 students divided into 3 small groups. It has been our experience that faculty can become overwhelmed with the amount of time guided reflective dialogue takes in order to make learning meaningful. Preparing for the seminar in advance by reviewing the stories helps us to keep the reflective dialogue from moving into a "feedback" session.

Critical conversations help students to move from *telling what they know* to *why they know*. Engaging learners in a critical dialogue also emphasizes the use of questions that fairly and respectfully challenge information. This type of question helps students to ignore unnecessary and irrelevant information and determine the aspects of the care situation that are significant. They assist students to reconstruct a situation, defend an action, hypothesize an expected consequence, identify values, and judge the appropriateness of an action.

## Faculty Guided Questions for Reflective Seminar:

- How did this make you feel? How did the patient make you feel?
- How did the patient feel about it? How do you know how the patient felt about it? (*Analysis* and evidence based *Inference*)
- What are the significant background details that contributed to this experience? (*Analysis* and *Inference*)
- How did these details influence your thinking?
- What sources of knowledge influenced/should have influenced your thinking? (*Interpretation* and *Explanation*)
- How have past experiences helped you to make sense out of the current situation?
- Do you think your feelings clouded the issue? Explain why or why not? (*Analysis* and *Explanation*)
- Describe what you were thinking about, as you were involved in the experience.
- What personal values or beliefs influenced your perspectives in this situation?
- What *may* have been taken for granted? (*Analysis* and preliminary *Inference*).
- What assumptions were made? (*Analysis* and *Inference*)
- What rationale was used to justify the assumptions? (*Interpretation* and *Explanation*)
- Were the assumptions correct? How do you know? (*Evaluation*)
- What things stand out for you as you reflect on this experience?
- What aspects of context impacted you and will help you to remember this experience? (*Analysis*, *Inference*, and *Explanation*)
- What were the consequences of your action? How could you have better dealt with the experience? What other choices did you have? (*Analysis, Inference, Explanation, Evaluation*)
- How has this had an impact on you? How will this experience impact your future practice? (*Inference* and *Explanation*)

**Figure 2: Guideline questions for the reflective seminar**

To assist with the process, as part of the seminar preparation, we provide our faculty a series of guided questions that they can use to enhance their dialogue skills with students. This prepared question list also helps faculty with conversations they have with students during the semester surrounding case studies or guiding students with reflective journaling. In Figure 2 we have included a question guideline that will be a good start for leading a reflective seminar. We use these questions as a general guideline ourselves, With experience teaching guided reflective seminars, you can expect to become comfortable in modifying the questions to closely fit the individual session as well as to plan when each questions is introduced.

Helping students to think critically about their clinical stories calls on faculty to use their own critical thinking skills well. One needs to interpret and analyze the student's story and draw accurate and meaningful inferences as to the probable meanings in the story in order to ask useful guided questions of the student. In time instructors become more adept at using their critical thinking skills in this way. Dialogue should be a critical conversation with students, guiding students thinking. In Figure 2 we have identified the critical thinking skills called into play when one of the guiding questions is asked, and so we can feel confident that we are practicing students in critical thinking when we ask these questions. Before beginning the seminar week, we make sure that we have secured the necessary time for the seminar, as guided reflection takes time!

**Teaching the lesson**

The reflective seminar is conducted at the end of the semester after the students' first clinical experience. Students' examine their experiences in the clinical setting using their critical thinking skills, connecting the theory they learned in the classroom to actual clinical practice. They meet in small seminar groups, each group taking place over a 3-hour period of time.

As the students begin to engage in their own clinical experiences, guided reflection becomes a more personal learning activity. Student's prepare for this activity by reflecting on their own clinical experiences and turn them into stories. Stories of their clinical experiences are then shared and discussed during the post clinical seminar. Using guided questions, like those outlined in Figure 2, faculty guide the students in a reflective dialogue to reinforce the learning connections the students are making and reinforce their use of critical thinking skills. Students document their learning insights into their story by creating a post-seminar reflection using the guided questions outlined in Figure 1.

This seminar exercise provides us insight into how best to train each individual student's clinical judgment skills. We can assess both how they applied clinical knowledge to the case at hand and their strength in using critical thinking skills.

Their responses to our seminar questions and their written reflections allowed us to examine what guided their thinking about the clinical case, and to see how they measured their personal learning accomplishments. Figure 3 is a short segment from one students' reflective journal.

> "One aspect of my clinical experience that left me with feelings of accomplishment was that at the end of my time with the patient, she thanked me and said I will be a wonderful nurse... encouraging her to continue her PT at home, increase her activity, and having her explain to me how she was going to manage her medical cares as well as emotional outlets while at home left me feeling like I helped this patient more when she was able to leave the hospital...[I was thinking]... what can I do now that will last when she is at home...The sources of knowledge that influenced my thinking was mainly that I tried to think of what was taught in class on patient education and interventions that would help her current status and help her in the future...I learned how to ask questions and get information in the way of a conversation and also to tell just enough about myself to gain their trust. I truly think this clinical experience has made a positive impact on me...I will keep in mind what I have learned for future practice."

### Feedback from the students

There are several aspects of this exercise that students find helpful for accomplishing their learning objectives. They have told us that the guided reflection gave them an opportunity to focus on their learning through clinical experience, and to think about what guided their nursing actions. The use of stories gave students an opportunity to share how their unique perspectives both aided and challenged their learning. Telling the stories in the seminar provided an opportunity for students to experience a sense of acceptance and support, and "brought nursing to life." Students indicated that sharing their stories and reflecting on and talking about their thinking and learning was an empowering experience. They also valued the opportunity to be intentional about analyzing their thinking (The practice of Metacognition) and making meaningful and evidence-based connections between their beliefs, prior knowledge and new knowledge. Students began to understand how critical thinking is evidenced in the context of real-life practice.

### Final comments on this example of teaching for thinking

While formal evaluation tools are necessary to assess learning (e.g. written care plans and exams), the use of students' stories provides a more personal perspective on their thinking and learning. The use of stories and the guided reflection offers a unique evaluation on the nature of their critical thinking skill, focusing specifically on the critical thinking skills of analysis and inference. While we have not stressed it strongly in this discussion, we also use this exercise to set our expectations for the critical thinking dispositions of open-mindedness and maturity, especially as it relates to clinical nursing practice (Facione and Facione, 2000). The use of stories gives students an opportunity to share their knowledge in unique ways, demonstrating tolerance for diverse points of view, and developing expertise in identifying a sound basis for making wise clinical decisions. Educators can capitalize on these stories by guiding conversations that help students' interpret their knowledge and achieve understanding of their actions.

Evaluating our own ability as nurse educators to think critically in the context of practice as we guide novice learners to develop their thinking is integral to the effectiveness of this classroom activity. Providing opportunities for nurse educators to share their own stories of their teaching and mentoring experiences enhances faculty awareness and sensitivity. As well, sharing their students' stories creates an opportunity to enhance their own knowledge about student thinking and a real awareness of diverse learners.

## References

Brookfield, S. Using Critical Incidents to Explore Learners' Assumptions. In J. M. a. Associates (Ed.), *Fostering critical reflection in adulthood: A guide to transformative and emancipatory learning.* (pp. 177-193). San Francisco: Jossey-Bass, Inc., 1990.

Brookfield, S. *Becoming a critically reflective teacher.* San Francisco: Jossey-Bass, Inc.

Brookfield, S. D. (2000). Transformative learning as ideology critique. In J. M. a. Associates (Ed.), *Learning as transformation: critical perspectives on a theory in progress.* San Francisco: Jossey-Bass Inc. , 1995.

Campbell, S. E. & Filer D. A. How can we continue to provide quality clinical education for increasing numbers of students with decreasing numbers of faculty? In M. Oermann, *Annual Review of Nursing Education: Vol. 6.* New York: Springer Publishing Company, 2008.

Campbell, S.& Dudley, K. (2005) Clinical Partner Model: Benefits for Education and Service, *Nurse Educator,* 30 (6), 271-274.

Carper, B. (1978). Fundamental patterns of knowing in nursing. *Advances in Nursing Science, 1*(1), 13-23.

Diekelmann, N. L., Ironside, P. M., & Harlow, M. Teaching practitioners of care: New pedagogies for the health professions. In N. Diekelmann & P. Ironside (Eds.), *Educating the Caregivers: Interpretive Pedagogies for the Health Professions* (Vol. 2, pp. 3-21). Madison, WI: University of Wisconsin Press, 2003.

Facione, P.A., Facione, N. C., & Giancarlo, CA, (2000). The Disposition toward critical thinking: Its character, measurement, and relationship to critical thinking skill. *Informal Logic* 20(1), 61-84.

Forneris, S. G. & Peden-McAlpine, C. (2007). *Evaluation of a reflective learning intervention to improve critical thinking in novice nurses. Journal of Advanced Nursing, 57(4), 410-421.*

Forneris, S. G. & Peden-McAlpine C.E. (2006). Contextual Learning: A reflective learning intervention for nursing education. *International Journal of Nursing Education Scholarship,* 3 (1), 1-18.

Forneris, S. (2004). Exploring the attributes of critical thinking: A conceptual basis. *International Journal of Nursing Education Scholarship, 1*(1), Article 9.

Ironside, P. M. (2003). New pedagogies for teaching thinking: The lived experiences of students and teachers enacting narrative pedagogy. *Journal of Nursing Education, 42*(11), 509-516.

Labov W. The transformation of experience in narrative syntax. In, Labov W. *Language in the Inner City: Studies in the Black English Vernacular*. Philadelphia, University of Pennsylvania Press, 1972.

Myrick, F. & Yonge, O. (2004). *Enhancing critical thinking in the preceptorship experience in nursing education. Journal of Advanced Nursing,* 45*(4), 371-380.*

Myrick, F., & Yonge, O. (2002). Preceptor questioning and student critical thinking. *Journal of Professional Nursing,* 18 (3), 176-181.

Peden-McAlpine, C., Tomlinson, P., Forneris, S. G., & Meyer, S. (2005). Evaluation of a reflective practice intervention to enhance family care. *Journal of Advanced Nursing, 49*(5), 494-501.

Reissman C. *Narrative Analysis.* Volume 30. Newbury Park, Sage Press, 1993.

# The Poster:
# A Critical Thinking and Creative Strategy in a Research Course

## *Joanne Profetto-McGrath & Karen Blumer Smith*

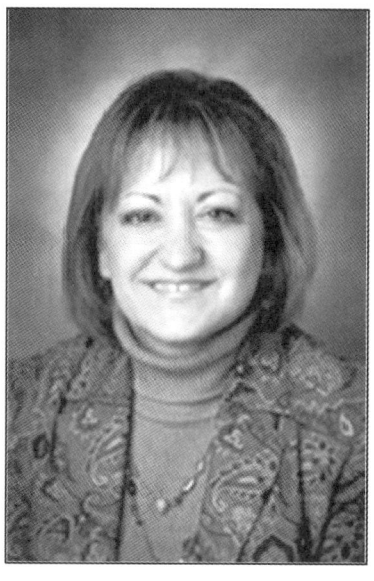

*Dr. Joanne Profetto-McGrath is Interim Dean at the Faculty of Nursing, at Canada's prestigious University of Alberta. She has been a scholar in the area of critical thinking throughout her career and we recommend her published data based discussions of strengthening the critical thinking skills of explanation and evaluation achieved by linking an evidence base with practice behavior. Dr. Profetto-McGrath's research program is well linked to her classroom and clinical teaching, for which she has been recognized for excellence on numerous occasions.*

*We had the pleasure of a personal meeting Dr. Profetto-McGrath on a visit to the University of Alberta's Evidence Based Practice Conference some years back. I am sure all those who attended recall the energy of that critical thinking community in contrast with the icy hush of those January snow-covered Edmonton nights.*

*Karen Blumer Smith is a research assistant on several of Profetto-McGrath's projects and a doctoral student mentee. Dr. Profetto-McGrath and Karen bring us this discussion of the use of a research poster to practice critical thinking skills and dispositions. The exercise offers a fine example of a teaching strategy that combines collaboration and competition in a context that emphasizes the practice of critical thinking skills..*

### The class session and the students

This group assignment was originally developed by Professor Profetto-McGrath for a required course in research methods as a way to enhance critical thinking skills while making research interesting, interactive, useful and fun. The course enrolled third year nursing students in a baccalaureate program and registered nurses in a two year baccalaureate completion program. The session would generalize to any health science course addressing the use of published research.

## The goal of the class session

The purpose of the lesson is to guide students (working in groups of 3 or 4) to retrieve, critique, and synthesize current research; to determine whether nursing practice at local agencies is congruent with the research findings; and to present their work in a clear manner using a poster format. The student groups communicate (translate/transfer) their work during in-class poster sessions.

There were number of purposes in mind in the creation of this assignment and all seemed attainable by coaching the students in the construction of a research poster. The course was intended to prepare students to retrieve published research studies that related to a specific and important health topic, phenomena or problem that has changed nursing practice.

## Learning Outcomes:

Students will demonstrate the ability to:

1) Interpret and analyze how research has changed practice in relationship to a specific health topic/phenomena/problem of interest.

2) Demonstrate critical thinking and creative skills using a poster medium.

3) Translate/transfer synthesized research knowledge from published studies to clinical practice.

The skills required for this assignment include prior exposure to reading research, some nursing knowledge, computer skills, library searching skills, group presentations skills and group process skills. The ability to use powerpoint or other presentation software is very helpful for this assignment. The completion of the assignment provides an additional opportunity to develop the above skills. The project also has the added potential to enhance collaboration and networking among nursing students and nurses in clinical practice settings.

## Focus for the course:

Research indicates that understanding, interpreting and incorporating research findings into practice is challenging for health care professionals. Some of these challenges include understanding and interpreting research, finding time to read the latest research findings, and indications that a preferred source of knowledge for nurses is social interaction. Posters are a quick way to present, analyze and understand current research findings. We recommend as good references on this topic the papers by Heye and Crowe (1996), Godkin (1999), and the two by Estabrooks and colleagues (2005a and 2005b) in the reference list below.

We assign this project to promote students' critical thinking skills through the use of appraisal skills relevant to the literature (interpretation, analysis, and evaluation), working collaboratively as a group to process the material and developing communication proficiency. The learning objectives are measured through our appraisal of the research posters and our assessment of the students' knowledge about the chosen research articles.

This assignment asks students to analyze nursing practice at local agencies, comparing what they observe at these agencies to the researched practices that they have located in the literature, and evaluating whether nursing practice at local agencies is congruent with the research findings. Part of this evaluation is the identification of examples of why the practice is supported by nursing research (or why not).

## Our work before the class for this assignment

Before the class begins, we prepare the following:

- List of practice topics related to their current clinical assignments that would be worthy of a research poster presentation.
- List of recently published research articles describing the preparation of a poster presentation (circulated in class or posted on the course Website).
- Handout outlining the guidelines for making and evaluating the poster.
- Group sign-up sheets for students to record their group name as well as each group member's name and contact information.
- Note-taking guide handout for students to use during class presentations related to the poster assignment.

## How this assignment is presented to students:

- During the course orientation, students learn that they will prepare posters working in small groups, and that the groups will be formed in Week 2 of the course. The assignment is then discussed during class time in week 2 as part of a lecture about poster presentations as a way to transfer/translate research findings into practice. We describe the components of a well done poster presentation,

Encourage them to use the note-taking guide to record information about the following questions raised in class drawn from the published articles included in the reference list:

- What is the purpose of the poster presentation assignment?
- What are the communication advantages of using a poster presentation?
- Why use a poster as opposed to another strategy/medium?
- What are the design elements for an effective poster presentation?
- How does a group effectively plan, develop and present the poster?

After the discussion of the poster presentation methodology, Dr. Profetto-McGrath explains the assignment using the guide prepared specifically for this purpose (Figure 1). Class time is used to acquaint the students with this assignment and encourage them to ask questions before they break into groups. We make it clear that they should contact us if they need more information or clarification.

To be sure that the students understand our expectations for the completed poster, we make available for students' viewing samples of posters completed by students in previous courses. To help them to get off on a good start with their group process we also share with students our expectations regarding group work and provide them with a brief overview of successful group process, including information about professionalism, group dynamics and respectful face-to-face and email communication.

Finally, we encourage the students to meet with us to review the research articles they have located before proceeding with the poster development. This part of the process is very helpful to students and necessary for the quality of the learning experience.

After a short question period, we explain the group tasks expected and ask each group to determine a group name that communicates something about their group. Having a group name promotes group identity and cohesion and seems to assist with the group process. We stress that group name should be professional and tasteful. For the remainder of the class session (15 to 20 minutes), students make plans to complete their group tasks. They assign a group liaison to facilitate their communication about the project. This person is responsible for communicating with the course instructor(s) when we ask for updates on the group's progress. Most of the work for this project occurs outside regular class time. The students have approximately 8 weeks to complete the assignment.

## FACULTY OF NURSING
## NURSING RESEARCH COURSE

### Group Assignment: Poster Presentation and Display

**Purpose of this assignment:**
- To identify how **research** related to a specific health topic/ phenomenon/clinical problem **has changed** *nursing practice*
- To demonstrate *critical thinking* and *creative skills* using a poster medium
- To communicate *synthesis* of nursing research in writing
- To enhance *collaboration* and *networking* among nursing students and nurses in clinical practice

These are your learning objectives for this assignment.

**Format:**
- Approximately 4 feet by 6 feet poster when assembled (poster should be portable, easy to assemble). The poster should be the students' own work, not that of a professional.
- A separate handout continuing a cover page, abstract and reference list must accompany the poster (APA Format)

**Poster components and content (Evaluation criteria):**
- Provide a purpose of the poster
- Provide a *brief history* of the health topic/phenomenon/problem
- *Define* **(describe and explain)** the topic/phenomenon/problem briefly
- Synthesize (analyze and evaluate) appropriate *nursing research* about the topic/phenomenon/problem and identify how this research has evolved (approximately 10-15 nursing research studies within last 10 years if applicable). **This is a major focus of poster.**
- Briefly describe how these findings are currently being used in nursing practice. Give concrete examples. You may wish to compare what is current practice at the institution where you are currently practicing or have practiced as compared to what is being written about in the literature
- Identify (analyze and explain) what *further research* needs to be conducted in order to fill existing gaps or to further extend the knowledge base related to the research topic/phenomenon/problem chosen. These may be worded in the form of questions or statements. Remember: Be specific.

**NOTE:**
☺ Poster guidelines and other important information will be provided in class
♦ Sample posters & pictures from previous groups' presentations will be available for viewing
➢ Time will be available in class for establishing groups & having a short initial meeting. Therefore it is VERY IMPORTANT that all students attend class

**\*Reference list** containing current information about developing and making posters and key research papers related to your health topic/practice problem**.**

**Figure 1: Guidelines for Poster Preparation and Presentation**

## What we expect from class participants

- We expect that this assignment might raise group process issues because the work necessitates consensus building and collaboration. We provide group members with an understanding of the dynamics of conflict resolution that might help groups deal with process issues. We model respect toward the students and expect the same behavior from student groups, reinforcing that this is a group assignment that they will receive a group mark.

- We expect quality presentations from the participants. We make this expectation apparent during the lecture.

- This assignment is designed to challenge and develop critical thinking skills. We have found that students often choose very difficult articles that prove to be challenging given their knowledge base and interpretive skills. Synthesizing them can be challenging. I encourage the groups to bring the articles to me with questions.

## The students' final work product - Poster Day

One option for poster presentation, useful if this work is part of an on-line lesson, is to have the student groups post their posters to a class website. However, having the student groups present their posters to their faculty and peers provides a stronger opportunity for improving students' critical thinking skills. The groups set up their posters along the perimeters of the classroom and present them to others in the class. The need to prepare for an effective presentation of the poster further assists them with synthesizing their learning and practices the critical thinking skills of analysis and explanation. During the in-class presentation, we move from group to group and discuss the posters with the students. Each group presents the poster for approximately 3-5 minutes. In presenting the poster session, we expect the students to articulate the research problem, purpose, and findings and how the particular research influences nursing practice. We pose two to three questions to the presenting group after the students have presented key aspects of their poster. The purpose of the questions is to stimulate a deeper interpretation of the material in the poster and to facilitate our evaluation of the student's critical appraisal skills, so the questions must be designed to stimulate higher level cognitive skills. This questioning process also serves as way to teach students how to ask higher level questions that reflect as well as stimulate others' critical thinking skills.

During the presentation week, we try to create an atmosphere of celebration, and as the instructors, we strive to make this session as informal and fun as possible so that our presence does not make the students too nervous. We also take pictures of the students and their posters for an album we keep to share during future course offerings.

Evaluations scores for the students' work are assigned later based on the criteria described in Figure 2, which is shared with the students when we introduced the assignment.

---

**Posters and content are evaluated based on the following components:**

- The overall visual presentation of the poster
- The presence of an identifiable purpose statement
- A brief history of the health topic/phenomena/problem
- A definition of the topic/phenomena/problem
- A reference list with approximately 10-15 recent research articles submitted together with the poster that indicates how the research relevant to the topic/phenomena/problem has evolved over time
- An explanation of how these findings are currently being *used in practice*. (For example, students might compare current practice at the institution where they are currently practicing or have practiced to what is reported as recommended practice in the literature
- A list of additional *nursing research* that needs to be conducted in order to fill existing gaps or to further extend the knowledge base related to the nursing research topic/phenomena/problem chosen. These can be written in the form of questions or statements.

**Presentation skills are evaluated based on:**
- The group's understanding of the research
- The group's ability to communicate findings clearly and concisely;
- Demonstrated professionalism: as indicated by speech, movement and body language during the presentation;
- Evidence of critical thinking skills: as demonstrated by their ability to answer questions posed by peers and instructor.

---

**Figure 2: Evaluation Rubric for the Poster Presentation Project**

We have used this assignment several times over the past ten years and we have received very positive feedback from students. Students have reported that while this assignment is labour intensive, they found it to be creative, fun, challenging, a great learning experience, and most of all an excellent way to enhance their critical thinking skills.

The value of the assignment extends outside the classroom to our academic and practice community. Each year several of the best posters are exhibited throughout the Faculty of Nursing building so that other students, educators, and members of the public can learn from the work done by students. One year, the posters from the course were part of a Faculty of Nursing's internal competition. The top three posters chosen by an independent committee received book and cash prizes. Staff at local agencies who were visited by students during the preparation of their posters asked students to bring the posters to the agency for viewing after they presented them in class. The staff requested these posters as a means to inform staff about nursing research relevant to their practice area. As a result these posters have served as a method to educate nurses in practice about the latest research.

## References

Block, S. M. (1996). Do's and don'ts of poster presentation. *Biophysical Journal*, 71(6), 3527-3529.
Butz, A. M., Kohr, L., & Jones, D. (2004). Developing a successful poster presentation. *Journal of Pediatric Health Care*, 18(1), 45-48.
Campbell, R. S. (2004). How to present, summarize, and defend your poster at the meeting. *Respiratory Care,* 49(10), 1217-1221.
Chabeli, M. M. (2002). A poster presentation as an evaluation method to facilitate reflective thinking skills in nursing education. *Curationis,* 25(3), 10-18.
Dumas, M. A., Gallo, K., & Shurpin, K. M. (1996). Research presentations: Disseminating knowledge for practice. *Journal of the American Academy of Nurse Practitioners*, 8(6), 277-281.
Englehart, N. (2004). Giving effective presentations. *Canadian Operating Room Nursing Journal,* 22(1), 22-24.
Estabrooks, C. A., Rutakumwa, W., O'Leary, K. A., Profetto-McGrath, J., Milner, M., & Levers, M. J. et al. (2005a). Sources of practice knowledge among nurses. *Qualitative Health Research*, 15(4), 460-476.
Estabrooks, C.A., Chong, H., Brigidear, K. & Profetto-McGrath, J. (2005b). Profiling Canadian nurses' preferred knowledge sources for clinical practice. *Canadian Journal of Nursing Research*, 37(2), 118-140.
Godkin, M.D. (1999). Posters meet clinical news needs. *Reflections* 25(3), 31.
Jackson, K., & Sheldon, L. (1998). Poster presentation: How to tell a story. *Paediatric Nursing*, 10(9), 36-37.
Maltby, H. J., & Serrell, M. (1998). The art of poster presentation. *Collegian: Journal of the Royal College of Nursing, Australia*, 5(2), 36-37.
Miracle, V. A. (2003). How to do an effective poster presentation in the workplace. *DCCN - Dimensions of Critical Care Nursing,* 22(4), 171-172.
Moule, P., Judd, M., & Girot, E. (1998). The poster presentation: What value to the teaching and assessment of research in pre-and post-registration nursing courses? *Nurse Education Today*, 18(3), 237-242.
Plouffe, D. A., & Koop, P. M. (2004). Constructing and presenting a poster: Instructions and some general principles. *Canadian Oncology Nursing Journal,* 14(2), 78-82.
Profetto-McGrath, J. (2003). The relationship of critical thinking skills and dispositions among baccalaureate nursing students. *Journal of Advanced Nursing, 43*(6), 569-577.
Profetto-McGrath, J. (2006). Critical thinking and evidence-based practice. *Journal of Professional Nursing, 21*(06), 364-371.
Profetto-McGrath, J., Hesketh, K., Lang, S., Estabrooks, C. (2003). A study of critical thinking and research utilization among nurses. *Western Journal of Nursing Research, 25*(3), 322-337.
Raymond, C., & Profetto-McGrath, J. (2005). Nurse educators' critical thinking: Reflection and Measurement. *Nursing Education in Practice*, 5, 209-217.
Vollman, K.M. (2005). Enhancing presentation skills for the advanced practice nurse. *AACN Clinical Issues* 16(1), 67-77.
Wharrad, J.J., Allcock, N. & Meal, A.G. (1995). The use of posters in the teaching of biological sciences on an undergraduate nursing course. *Nurse Education Today*, 15(5), 370-374.
White, A., & White, L. (2003). Preparing a poster. *Acupuncture in Medicine*, 21(1-2), 23-27.
Wipke-Tevis, D.D., & Williams, D.A. (2002). Preparing and presenting a research poster. *Journal of Vascular Nursing*, 20(4), 138-142.
Worrell, J., & Profetto-McGrath, J. (2007). Critical thinking as an outcome of context-based learning among post-RN students: A literature review. *Nurse Education Today, 27,* 420-426.

# Problem-Based Learning in a Competency-Based Medical Assistants Curriculum

## *Rodney L. Tomczak*

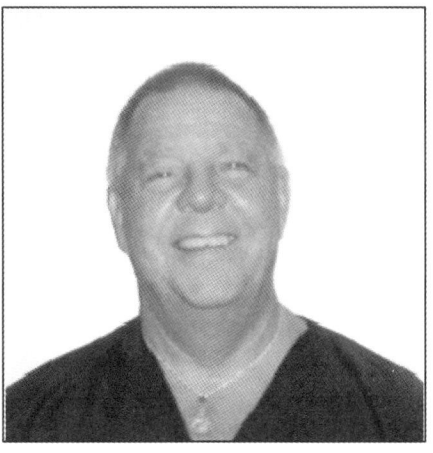

*We had the pleasure of meeting Professor Tomczak at the Inaugural Nova Southeastern University Conference on Critical Thinking and Clinical Judgment. Dr. Tomczak has been a professor of Podiatric Medicine and Surgery at Des Moines Medical University in Des Moines, Iowa, and a clinical professor at the Ohio State University Muscular Skeletal Institute in Columbus Ohio. He also holds a doctoral degree in Adult Education from Drake University. Currently he is the Chair of Education at Everest Institute, and co-chairman of the Problem-based learning curriculum for Ohio State University College of Medicine.*

*We know you will enjoy the lesson he is sharing here in this chapter, as well as the classic references on teaching and learning. Yes, there really is a reference here from the 1890 Journal 'Science.' Through the use of clinical scenarios he teaches phlebotomy students about the unexpected variation of problems that present in clinical practice. We see where training critical thinking is an integral part of training clinical expertise and sound clinical reasoning. Thank you, Dr. Tomczak, for your wonderful humor and for this creative problem-based learning exercise.*

### Background

There is a huge difference between hitting a baseball placed on a tee, something small children do, and hitting an 85 mph curve ball. One can easily stand in a batters' box and employ the same mechanics repeatedly and learn to hit that ball off the tee fairly consistently. Unfortunately, as one progresses through the athletic milieu, the variables such as speed and arc of the ball, psychological distractions like crowd noise, and topography of the batters' box change. Those who can't hit the curve under these evolving circumstances have no chance to make the major leagues.

In the television show *Star Trek* there was constant psychological tension and hermeneutic disequilibrium between Spock and Kirk. Strict Aristotelian logic versus Kohler's Problem Solving by insight was the underlying theme of most shows. Today, on the TV show *House, MD*, we are treated to the problem-solving skills of Gregory House, MD whose skills are more often than not met with dire consequences and the drama of pulling a patient back from the grasp of death, until another trial and error attempt is made to salvage a soul.

Teaching in the Allied Health Profession is often moving tortuously slow toward a terminal behavior, step by step along a path which at times does not even allow binary decisions. The trainer inches the student along a path toward successful completion of a task, say drawing venous blood from the antecubital space of the elbow. There is no deviation. There's probably only miniscule differences between the way it's done in New York and the way it's performed in San Francisco. Move along in the training process too quickly and mistakes occur and the student reverts to trial and error behavior. Move too slowly and the quick graspers become bored. The steps are always the same, prepare the equipment, make a preliminary choice of a target vein, apply the tourniquet…

I have this friend, a surgeon who was very well trained. I know this is true because I had the same training. I've trained many surgeons and have come to the conclusion I could train an ape or robot to perform most procedures. Why? As long as there are no creative decisions to be made, the process of surgery is rather straight forward and as long as the procedure is broken down into step by step tasks, it really is relatively straight forward. More complicated procedures simply mean more steps…unless something goes wrong. Then, problem solving and higher order thinking skills come into play. Now you have to hit that 90 mph curve ball in Yankee Stadium in the ninth inning of the seventh game of the World Series.

My friend never enjoyed operating after completing his residency. The thought of something going wrong terrified him and when it did, he had to actually go sit down in the corner and try and think his way through the problem. He was unpracticed and uncomfortable with the process of problem solving. He eventually quit surgery and went into administration. He couldn't hit the curve ball.

## Class Session and Students

A successful Medical Assistant Program has consisted of shaping a number of terminal behaviors, perhaps the most invasive and complicated being phlebotomy. Students vary in age from post high school to adults with grown children. Ninety-five percent of the students are female.

Surgical Interns are initially exasperated by their own fumbling and erratic performance in tying surgical knots. According to the Fitts and Posner model of motor skills acquisition (Fitts & Posner, 1967), this evolves into integration and automation. This automation is best characterized by the late night scenario where the intern is reading while ambidextrously tying surgical knots without paying attention to the motor skill. Medical assistant students do not enjoy the luxury of constant repetition, so a virtual reality arm model with "antecubital veins" is employed for multiple practice opportunities.

Practice makes perfect when there are no variables, and this is the case with the simple mechanics of tying knots. But the human condition is rarely constant, so trying to teach the variables of venipuncture with a model which does not change is the challenge. We need to teach students to hit the curve balls of venipuncture.

The challenge for the professor is to identify these changing variables in venipuncture, and to place them in a problem-based learning scenario which fosters solutions within a clinical context without violating the diagnosis taboo, and yet still allowing for on the spot assessment. One way to have students identify these variables is to guide them to think through the scenario. Major questions to be asked during the scenario include:

1. "What do you think has happened?"
2. "Why do you think this has happened?"
3. "What will you do to fix it?"
4. "What would you do differently next time?"

Notice that Question 2 asks for reason giving, an important expectation to train for accountability of practice and a way to practice the critical thinking skills of analysis, inference and evaluation. Question 4 targets these three critical thinking skills as well.

Rather than present only one scenario, I offer three examples of the use of clinical scenarios to train critical thinking skills in the performance of phlebotomy. Each asks students to apply anatomy and physiology principles and venipuncture technique, but the patient management problems force the students

*224 Critical Thinking and Clinical Reasoning in the Health Sciences: A Teaching Anthology*

to confront unexpected clinical events that require critical thinking and competent clinical judgment.

# PROBLEM I

**Information for Instructors:** There is a movement in the phlebotomy community to use blood pressure cuffs rather than a thin stretchable band for a tourniquet to cause venous engorgement but allow arterial inflow while performing the blood draw. In an individual with a narrow pulse pressure, or low blood pressure, there is a small margin of error between venous engorgement and complete arterial occlusion.

**Scenario** *(this information is given to the student)***:** The physician who you are working for instructs you to use a blood pressure cuff for a phlebotomy on a 25 year old, female, latex allergic patient because all tourniquets in the office happen to contain latex. As the vacuum tube is pushed into the needle, there is a "blood flash" which quickly diminishes to no more flow. Your attempts to reposition the needle are futile.

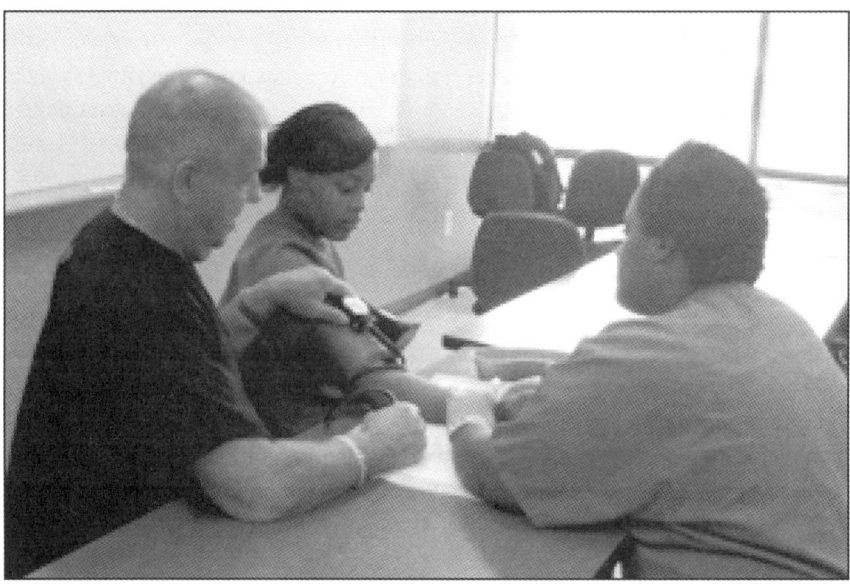

**Problem prompt:** What is your assessment of the problem and plan of action? Here is where the questions above come into play:
       1. "What do you think has happened?"
       2. "Why do you think this has happened?"
       3. "What will you do to fix it?"
       4. "What would you do differently next time?"

## Process for Problem I

Students can either work individually or in groups on these problems, in class or at home. My goal is to provide them time to evolve some hypotheses about what may be going wrong, and to assess the strength of these hypotheses, resolving the problem of why the blood sample is not forthcoming. This process of allowing for multiple working hypotheses has been known to foster growth in thinking for at least as long ago as 1890 when it was advocated by Chamberlin. Students are expected to feel Piagetian disequilibrium and will want to just be told the answer. Teachers may think it is more efficient to merely tell the students that the blood flow has been occluded by the cuff pressure, but learning this fact within the context of a patient problem makes retrieval of the information much more accessible (Bruner, 1961), and future curve balls become easier to hit.

This problem actually concerns the medical assistant's mechanics in relation to the patient's blood pressure. The medical assistant is using a new mechanism, a blood pressure cuff, which may be over inflated and completely occluding blood flow. Unless the cuff is immediately released, there may be no more flow through the vein into the tube. Release of the valve and deflation of the cuff requires significant manual dexterity when performed with one hand while the other hand is cradling the test tube. It is more complicated than a simple rubber strap which can be released with a simple tug on a free end of the tourniquet. The first question which arises is whether the phlebotomist completely released the blood pressure cuff, an action which requires more dexterity than removing a stretchable tourniquet. On the other hand, the phlebotomist may have punctured completely through the vein or repositioned the needle such that blood flow is halted. Phlebotomists are taught a sequence of actions which should be routinely followed. When blood flow ceases, the needle should be readjusted if the tourniquet has already been released.

The four questions can be asked after the students have some time to digest the problem. Should the scenario occur in "real time" as a blood draw is underway on another student, it is inappropriate to start asking hypothetical questions about what happened. Ironically, this is the opportunity for instructors to use their own problem solving skills to correct the complication which is occurring before their eyes and turn it into a "teaching moment." This usually happens after the needle is removed from the student-patient donor.

This is an example of an ill-defined problem with little chance of immediately vectoring to a one and only correct answer. As a result, there are multiple avenues for discussion and hypotheses.

## PROBLEM II

**Information for Instructor:** Medical Assistants may be required to draw blood from a patient whose medical history and present medications are unfamiliar. Patients such as this could be on platelet or anti-coagulation therapy. If routine chemistries or CBC are ordered, the medical assistant drawing blood may not be aware of the potential for hemorrhage.

**Scenario:** You are asked to draw blood from a 65 year old male for serum electrolytes. After filling the red top tube, you remove the needle from the patient, apply pressure with a cotton ball, and then ask the patient to continue applying pressure while you prepare the tube for transport. Before applying an adhesive bandage, you remove the cotton ball and discover a marble sized hematoma has already formed at the puncture sight. What is your assessment and plan of action?

The same questions work to draw out student's thinking for this problem situation, but in a different order:
1. "What do you think has happened?"
2. "What will you do to fix it?"
3. "Why do you think this has happened?"
4. "What would you do differently next time?"

**Process for Problem II**

The process for this scenario is the same as for Problem 1, individual or group work that allows students time to form hypotheses about the nature of the problem, to seek additional information and move in the direction of the action needed to resolve the unexpected clinical event. This problem involves the immediate assessment of hematoma formation, and regardless of the cause, the student is expected to prevent further hemorrhage. This is an example of the necessity of being able to think accurately and rapidly in an unfamiliar situation, processing information as quickly as possible and adapting to the unknown.

Failure would to be to run for the physician without adequate pressure being applied to the venipuncture site. Students immediately want to make the hematoma "go away" as if to correct an error on their part. This can't be done. Laying blame is not the issue here. The hematoma is likely extravascular and although somewhat startling initially, with the proper treatment, it will resolve.

The "why this happened" is not the first consideration. After the hemorrhaging is stopped the analysis of how the problem originated can be addressed, and a plan for the next time can be designed. Should every patient be asked about medication? Should the ordering physician let the phlebotomist know if there is anti-coagulation therapy? Or, should every patient be treated as if they have a tendency to hemorrhage? Fully debriefing this clinical scenario, and fully exploring each of these potential protocol changes for the reasons supporting each, is an exercise that trains critical thinking skills (analysis, inference, explanation, and evaluation) and nurtures the disposition to be concerned about anticipating the consequences of high stakes judgments (analyticity).

## PROBLEM III

**Information for Instructor:** In this scenario a blood drawer accidentally sticks herself with a needle contaminated with a patient's blood and in so doing instantly becomes a new patient. For the purpose of this scenario, let us assume that Universal Precautions were taken, but nonetheless this incident occurred. In a moment of crisis such as this, the algorithm for action is often forgotten. I know from personal experience and even after 25 years in the OR, it takes the circulating nurse to calmly initiate the proper protocol and assuage my panic.

In addition to training the students in thinking well about the scenario, a review and improved understanding of the 'why' of the proper follow-up procedures are the goals of this problem.

**Scenario:** After completing an exceptionally difficult blood draw during which the patient squirmed and cried, you accidentally stick yourself with the contaminated needle while trying to engage the safety mechanism. What should you do? Once again the four questions all are important.
   1. "What do you think has happened?"
   2. "What will you do to fix it?"
   3. "Why do you think this has happened?"
   4. "What would you do differently next time?"


### Process for Problem III

This is a complicated problem. Using the recommended four questions to externalize students' thinking about this scenario helps the instructor to assess how well students have learned key information in this most important content area. Although the event is well defined in causation, its occurrence calls for a myriad of possible actions and at best a delayed resolution. My learning objectives for this session include OSHA/HIPPA issues, an exploration of the issues surrounding the patient's willingness to be tested for communicable diseases, the possibility of infectious disease prophylaxis, and the discussion about responsibilities toward the phlebotomist's sexual partner. The scenario offers the opportunity to examine the problem in a context of uncertainty. What action must be taken before the definitive exclusion of potential disease?

## Conclusion

Even among the most seasoned health care professionals, this scenario is carried out on a daily basis around the world. There is a certain assumption of risk which all health care providers who come in contact with bodily fluids must assume. Although the potential for infection is rare, it does exist. For this reason this scenario is particularly useful for training practicing clinicians in all health science fields.

## SUMMARY THOUGHTS

I prefer to use this method in the context of problem-based <u>learning</u> rather than problem-based <u>testing</u>. This model serves as a tool to help integrate decision making and problem recognition and resolution into the health professions. Students still perform well on standard multiple-choice tests if the learning process is supplemented with problem- or case-based learning. There should be no fear that "fact transfer time" is diminished by allowing students to think about situations they may encounter which can not be routinely taught in a classroom or laboratory where simulations are constant and non-variable.

Testing in a competency based problem-based learning curriculum presents a unique set of challenges. Problem-based learning gained its North American foothold at McMaster University in Hamilton, Ontario under the guidance of Howard Barrows, MD a trained neurologist. The original cohort of 20 medical students in 1969 were not subjected to conventional testing but were evaluated through an ongoing subjective process (Neufeld & Barrows, 1974). It wasn't until 1991 that the personal progress index examination was introduced at McMaster to emphasize to students that, irrespective of the enjoyment of learning in tutorial, the acquisition of a progressively sophisticated medical knowledge base was required for successful graduation from the program (Neville & Norman, 2007).

Malcolm Knowles, the father of adult education, felt a disdain for testing adult learners. He thought that since adults were self-motivated, there was no need for testing (Knowles, Holton & Swanson, 2005). Barrows felt the same way about self-motivation and self-directed learning skills relying more on self-assessment than testing (Barrows, 1986). We are easily able to assess clinical competencies throughout the curriculum at Everest Institute in Columbus, but the assessment of didactic information in a student-directed problem-oriented conceptual fashion, along with judging a student's ability to handle complications, is more difficult.

Not everyone has joined the problem-based learning method of education. Some prominent medical educators discern multiple practical and philosophical problems with problem-based learning and have not gotten on board (Shanley, 2007). Testing is one of the major problems. The multiple choice high stakes exam is still the bench mark for didactic knowledge and certification. Problem solving skills are rarely evaluated in the Medical Assistant's world.

The oral examinations we used in the Problem-based curriculum in Des Moines relied heavily on subjective evaluations. As a result, grades were assigned as "Pass" or "Fail." At Ohio State we used a serial written test where students would complete one section, then turn it in. They would then be given the answers to the first section with additional questions to be answered. This continued a few more times until problem resolution. Students were required to use their critical thinking skills and the fund of knowledge they had learned during the quarter to successfully solve the sequential clinical management problems.

Complications of venipuncture are extremely difficult to examine uniformly on phlebotomy models. These models don't exhibit life like responses, and some complications cannot be modeled or practiced. We couldn't, for instance, ask a surgical resident to nick a renal artery to see how he or she responds. We can work through this complication and the correct response in a conference and only hope it never occurs. The same goes for phlebotomy mistakes. We can only pose the problem and then ask:

1. "What do you think has happened?"
2. "What will you do to fix it?"
3. "Why do you think this has happened?"
4. "What would you do differently next time?"

Routine tasks performed on a daily basis by medical assistants can achieve a type of automation, like hitting that baseball off a tee, but, when the situations change and complications arise, medical assistants must be able to adapt. A lecturer can cover multiple facts, but placing the learning objectives of a lecture within the context of a patient problem allows the student something to hang facts on. It makes them not only more meaningful, but also more retrievable. Research that explores the storage of information as episodic memory probably explains why it is that we are better able to retain information learned in the context of a case scenario (Slovic, Frishoff, & Lichtenstein, 1977).

Patient problems also offer the student the opportunity to constantly reassess thoughts and actions and consider if they might have done something different to improve the outcome. Teachers sometimes fear their own proficiency at conducting these sessions, but beginning with a case presentation and entertaining feedback with the same four questions listed earlier will facilitate implementation of problem-based learning into a lecture-based curriculum. There is no right or wrong way to facilitate problem-based learning. As long as the instructor uses a bit of imagination or real life experiences as a basis to build a case, the students will gain critical thinking skills.

## References

Barrows, H. S. (1986). A taxonomy of problem-based learning methods. Medical Education, 20, 481-486.
Bruner, J. S. (1961). The Act of Discovery, *Harvard Educational Review*, 31(1), 21-32.
Chamberlin, T. C. (1890). The Method of Multiple Working Hypotheses. *Science*, 15, 92-97.
Fitts, PM, Posner, MI. *Human Performance,* Belmont, CA, Brooks/Cole, 1967.
Knowles, M.S., Holton, E.F. III & Swanson, R. A. *The Adult Learner.* 6th Ed. Burlington, MA: Elsevier, 2005.
Neufeld, V.R. & Barrows, H. S. (1974). The "McMaster Philosophy:" an approach to medical education. *Journal of Medical Education*. 49, 1040-1050.
Neville, A.J. & Norman, G.R. (2007). PBL in the undergraduate program at McMaster university: three iterations in three decades. *Academic Medicine,* 82 (4), 370-374.
Shanley, P.F. (2007). Leaving the "Empty Glass" of problem-based learning behind: new assumptions and a revised model for case study in pre-clinical education. Academic Medicine, 82, 479-485.
Slovic, P., Frishoff, B. & Lichtenstein, S. (1977). Behavioral decision theory. *Annual Review of Psychology*, 28, 1-39.

*Here are a few additional papers on teaching for thinking by Dr. Tomczak:*

Tomczak, R. (1990). The Podiatric Medical Student as an Adult Learner, *The Journal of Current Podiatric Medicine,* 39, 25,..
Tomczak, R. (1993). Toward a Philosophy of Podiatric Medical Education, *Journal of the American Podiatric Medical Association,* 42, 83.

# Using Theoretical Foundations for a Community Health Nursing or a Population Health Course

## Caroline R. Ellermann

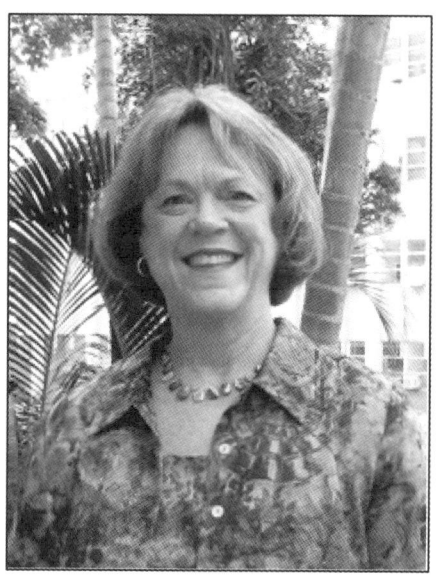

*Dr. Ellermann teaches at Northern Arizona University, Flagstaff, in the School of Nursing. We came to know her through her work in using logic models to stimulate critical thinking in health science students. She began to develop this interest while teaching undergraduate and graduate nursing students at the University of Hawaii at Manoa, United States.*

*This lesson applies well supported theoretical models to inform the analysis of a community health study and to design a modest intervention that could be carried out by a student intern during a clinical rotation. It is written for senior nursing students, but its applicability for students in other branches of the health sciences is obvious. This lesson is a fine example of the value theoretical models to inform practice. We like the idea of bringing the models to the students, as this type of exercise too often frustrates baccalaureate level students unnecessarily when they are asked to find relevant theoretical models for themselves. Students and clinicians alike will be more likely to seek out relevant models after experiencing this exercise, bridging another theory-practice gap.*

### The class session and the students

I teach this lesson to students in two programs: public health and community health nursing. The course is a senior seminar that includes a group project where students carry out a focused assessment of a specific community, and design a primary prevention intervention that addresses one deficit in the health of that community. This class occurs early in the semester, and provides a foundation to support the community assessment and the selection of the intervention.

Working in groups of two or three, students conduct the community assessment by gathering and analyzing community health data, by interviewing and learning from key informants in the community, and through their own personal observation of the community. I work with each group of students individually to be sure that they are conducting a sound analysis of the community's health problems and are conducting the community assessment in a professional manner. As a part of the project, students consult with a local Public Health District Supervisor in the selection of the specific socio-geo-political and/or aggregate community and the specific health issue or topic.

The community assessment process is taught in different sessions of this course. Figure 1 summarizes this assignment, and structures the paper reporting the work that is required for completion of the course. Each student in the group examines a different aspect of the health problem and contributes an individual community action plan. I ask students to identify both short and long term outcomes in their action plan, and I hold them accountable for carrying out the short term outcomes. This initial community work must be conceived, implemented and completed within about two months and often involves building partnerships in the community that can later be used to address the long term outcomes as well.

An evaluation component is also a necessary piece of the action plan. They must think about how they would measure the impact of their community interactions and the achievement of the outcomes that they intend to influence or control.

**The goal of this class session**

The goal for this class is for students to understand how to organize and frame their thinking about promoting health in populations from a theory-based perspective. Integrating multiple modes of critical thinking is essential for success in the assigned project. Students need to understand the rationale for selecting a guiding frame, to identify potential relevant guiding theories, to know how to obtain appropriate community evidence for the selected perspective, to decide on options, to understand the influence of context, and to evaluate how the information is linked. In addition, it is important that the students understand the domain specific-knowledge of population care and specifically, working with communities.

**Guidelines for conducting a community assessment**

1. Initiate your assessment by completing a windshield survey (tour of the census area), remembering to look for clues (data) related to the specific health issue in your assigned community.

2. Collect statistical data, epidemiological trends data, and interviews of community leaders and key informants (PHN, clinic staff, neighborhood board members, policy makers, shop owners, police, fireman, educators and so on, as is relevant to your topic).

3. Determine why the health issue is relevant to your assigned community. Include health status indicators and comparisons of local community to regional, county, state, national and/or world trends. Utilize classic and current data.

4. Seek evidence from the published literature to explain positive and negative influences of the specific health issue under investigation on the health of populations.

5. Apply a theoretical model that is appropriate to the specific health issue under investigation to analyze your community and explain your assessment.

6. In light of your completed assessment, consider specific long term and short term goals for improvement of the specific health issue in your community.

7. Provide an action plan that addresses all of the community weaknesses for the health issue and includes an evaluation module.

Figure 1: Guideline for Community Health Assessment

The class session addresses the analysis of impact of various factors on the health of populations, and the synthesis of theory and evidence-based research to guide an intervention to enhance the health of populations. By the end of this class session students should have gained enough skill in applying theoretical models to select a model to guide their own community assessment project.

## Learning objectives:

By listening to the class presentation, and reviewing and evaluating various theoretical models presented in class, students will be able to:

1. Explain how the use of theoretical models provides varying perspectives on a community health assessment (analysis and explanation).

2. Analyze and compare the utility of various theoretical models for use in population care (interpretation and analysis).
3. Identify and integrate appropriate community health related data to support an accurate community health analysis (analysis and inference).
4. Apply a logic model to relevant community data and analyze the information gained from the model in terms of the evaluation of a primary prevention intervention (analysis and evaluation).

**The actual materials used for the class session:**

Eight to ten theoretical or conceptual models currently in use in the health sciences are pre-selected for students to evaluate. The models must be available for use in the class session, so I prepare small packets that include these models before class. I select a variety of different models that take varying perspectives and range across a variety of outcomes when they are applied to a community assessment. When selecting the models for this exercise it is essential to anticipate the kinds of projects your students will be preparing so that at least one model can be successfully applied to their community health issue during this class session. For example, I know that there will be students who will design a final intervention project related to health promotion, so I include a health promotion model in the packets. I also know that students may seek to improve the functional health care delivery system in their chosen community, so consequently, one or more systems models should be in the packet. The graphic representation of the model, a brief description of the model, and a discussion of how it is used to describe, explain or predict community health issues, can be found in texts or prepared from published theory papers. Ideally the students will have some exposure to many of the models in the packet prior to being asked to apply them in this exercise, but the packet is a shortcut to retrieving applicable models and allows class time to be used for the application of the models and intervention planning.

Examples of appropriate models that I use for my nursing and public health students include: the Green and Kreuter Precede-Proceed Model for Health Promotion Planning and Evaluation (1991); Pender's Health Promotion Model (1996); King's General Systems Framework (1971, George, 2002); Neuman's Health Systems Model (1994); Becker's Health Beliefs Model (1974; Janz & Becker, 1984); Anderson and McFarlane's Community-as-Partner Model (1996); W. K. Kellogg Foundation logic model (2004); Green's Ecological Model (1992); Stokols Ecological Model (1992); and Watson's Carative Model (1985). Most of these models are well known, but I have included a reference for each at the end of this chapter. As you might already be thinking, some of these models are more useful than others. Discerning which of the models provide value is a large part of the class exercise.

**How I teach this lesson:**

This class session has two sections, the first is a lecture where I discuss the importance of using theoretical models to analyze community health problems and plan community health interventions, and a second section where students begin to examine theoretical models that can help them to carry out a community assessment and design a community intervention plan. This class is intended to assure that they will do a systematic analysis and use research based models to intervene for improvement in public health.

I begin the lecture by introducing the metaphor of a kaleidoscope to visually illustrate the point that the answers you get when assessing a community depend on the view taken of the community. For example, I explain that if one looks for health beliefs using a health belief model, they will gain an understanding of the collective health beliefs, attitudes and values that influence the populations' life choices and subsequent health. But the Health Belief Model will not be particularly helpful for understanding the influence of context on community health. For examining how people are situated I the community, they would be better served by using an ecologically focused model. And so on.

I next review the application of a theoretical model, highlighting the inherent benefit of this systematic method of assessing or explaining health. I also discuss the added potential benefit of using an appropriate theory to guide practice. In this part of the class I want to be sure that students grasp the fact that established theoretical models have consistent logical links that have typically been supported through research. For population health a useful practice model 1) applies to multiple levels of clients, 2) addresses health promotion, illness preventions or resolution of existing problems, and 3) provides directions for nursing activities to achieve goals of care.

Finally I take a few moments to discuss the utility of logic models. It is in this part of the session that I stress the important dimension of using critical thinking in problem identification and problem solving when assessing the health needs of a community. As a foundation, I describe logical models as useful for: 1) bringing details to broad goals, 2) illustrating if-then relationships or a chain of events, 3) identifying assumptions and gaps, and 4) summarizing complex events such that signals for evaluation points may become clearer.

In the second section of the class, students work together in their smaller clinical groups. I give them a guideline for this part of the discussion to assure that they have a good opportunity to meet the learning goals. Figure 2 briefly describes the guideline. The time available for this portion of the class can vary but I like to provide them at least 45 minutes to work down the suggested questions.

---

**Exploring the applicability of theoretical models to the project**

Briefly discuss each of the following questions in your small groups:

1. What models help to explain the health issue we've chosen?
2. Are we examining the health issue from a health prevention, health promotion, system analysis, or ecological frame?
3. Recalling the idea of 'kaleidoscope,' how do the different models provide differing perspectives on improving health in the community?
4. What model characteristics are most important?
5. What data must be gathered from the community?
6. Are we attempting to create future partnerships to stimulate an intervention?
7. What models relate to influences we think we need to change?

Your answers to these questions will determine your best choice of a theoretical model for your project.

---

**Figure 2: Identify an Appropriate Theoretical Model**

Initially the students dialogue about what constitutes a useful model. Most of these discussions culminate in the correct conclusion that the model must be focused on a desired outcome and the concepts must be relevant to the problem that will be addressed. They often will also identify 'clarity,' 'explanatory or predictive power,' or some other aspects of theory application in these discussions. Each member of the group has the model packet and can use these examples to think abstractly about why they seem to be useful (or not). In the course of the discussion, the group begins to zero in on a few of the models as more applicable for potential use. I walk around from group to group to reinforce good thinking and also to help assure that each group moves on to address all the questions on the list in the time available.

The question "which data would need to be gathered from a community" takes on varying appearances, depending on the variety of the variables included in the models the students have identified as relevant. The intent is for students to begin to think about the multi-dimensional aspects of populations that influence health. I'm hoping that they will generalize this insight when they initiate their clinical assignment, refining and relying on patterns of thinking that have been stimulated and practiced in this classroom exercise. By examining potentially relevant models and thinking about potentially relevant data in a small group discussion, students are more likely able to identify needed data when they work individually or in groups out in the community.

## The student work product

Later in the course, all of the student groups complete their community assessment. Each group member details a different aspect of the community health problem, identifying a weakness, analyzing the relevant data, applying an appropriate model and developing an action plan for that specific weakness. Each student writes an individual paper reporting this work.

Additional faculty-student discussions are required to continue the multi-dimensional critical thinking necessary to complete this project. However, students are able to logically link the data that they gather during the community assessment, to identify a deficit, and finally to structure an appropriate measurable outcome. Collected data, detailed community strengths and weaknesses, and recommended actions are shared with the public health officials responsible for the community. While the students do not carry out the proposed actions themselves, actions are often taken based on the student assessment.

## Project evaluation

Understanding and interpretation of the assignment is evaluated in a graded paper. In terms of this class session, I evaluate the application of the theoretical models for organizational adequacy, and for appropriately placed community data within a selected frame, of sufficient collection of data for intervention decision making, and finally, for developing and implementing a logical intervention that is supported by the community data and the theoretical model chosen to guide the project.

> My guideline for this paper covers the following expectations:
> 1) Show evidence of a comprehensive socio-geo-political assessment
> 2) Identify and discuss relevant health related strengths and weaknesses within the community
> 3) Briefly explain why strengths and weaknesses exist in the community
> 4) Develop a measurable action plan to address a specific weakness
> 5) Reference appropriate theoretical model(s)

Requiring consistency between community data, descriptive and predictive models and a measurable action plan exercises these senior students' critical thinking skills (analysis, inference and evaluation) in an authentic community health problem frame.

**Student feedback and some final thoughts**

I caution students that graphic representations of their chosen theories only depict estimations of reality, but are not reality. Similarly the data gathered will never completely reflect all aspects of the community. Options excluded by these selection processes may have influenced the results of the exercise and may not provide all that nurses really want to know. The models will also not provide them an assurance that the planned interventions will make a true difference, only a well analyzed intervention plan grounded in evidence based inference.

Students find the approach a new way to organize their thinking about outcomes of care. Because many of the ideas are highly theoretical, it often takes weeks of the students' delving into their clinical community assessment project and planning the intervention before the 'Ah-ha!' moment comes. It is only near the end of the project that students begin to understand the idea of the 'kaleidoscopic view.' They begin to see that their work product results from analyzing the problems of their community using the specific models that they have chosen, considering several possible paths, selecting a route, and then committing to working toward a final outcome.

**References**

Anderson, E.T. & McFarlane, J. *Community as Partner: Theory and Practice in Nursing.* Philadelphia: Lippincott, 1996.

Becker, M.H. (1974). The health belief model and personal health behavior. *Health Education Monograph,* 2, 324–508.

Ellermann, C.R., Kataoka-Yahiro, M. R. & Wong, L.C. (2006). Logic models used to enhance critical thinking. *Journal of Nursing Education,* 45(6), 220-226.

Green, L. W. & Kreuter, M. W. *Health Promotion Planning: An Educational and Environmental Approach,* 2$^{nd}$ Ed. Mountain View, CA: Mayfield Publishing Company, 1991.

Green, L.W. (1992). The health promotion research agenda revisited. *American Journal of Health Promotion,* 6, 411-413.

Janz, N.K. & Becker, M.H. (1984). The Health Belief Model a Decade Later. *Health Education Quarterly,* 11(1), 1-47.

King, I. *Toward a Theory For Nursing* John Wiley & Sons, Inc: New York, 1971.

King, I. M. Systems framework and theory of goal attainment. In J. B. George, (Ed.) *Nursing Theories: The Base for Professional Nursing Practice,* 5$^{th}$ Ed., (pp.241-268). Upper Saddle River, NJ: Prentice Hall, 2002.

Neuman, B. *The Neuman Systems Model* , 3$^{rd}$ Ed. Norwalk, CT: Appleton & Lange, 1994.

Neuman, B. The Neuman Systems Model. In, J. B. George (Ed). *Nursing Theories: The Base for Professional Nursing Practice,* 5$^{th}$ Ed. (pp, 339-384). Upper Saddle River, NJ: Prentice Hall, 2002.

Pender, N.J. *Health Promotion in Nursing Practice*, 3rd Ed.. Stamford, CT: Appleton & Lange, 1996.
Stokols, D. (1992). Establishing and maintaining healthy environments: Toward a social ecology of health promotion. *American Psychologist*, 47, 6-22.
Watson, J. *Nursing: The Philosophy and Science of Caring*. Boulder, CO: Co Associated University Press, 1985.
Kelley, J.H. & Johnson, B. Theory of Transpersonal caring: Jean Watson. In, J. B. George, (Ed.). *Nursing Theories: The Base for Professional Nursing Practice,* 5th Ed. (pp. 339-384). Upper Saddle River NJ: Prentice Hall, 2002.
W. K. Kellogg Foundation (2004). *Logic Model Development Guide*. Battle Creek, MI:

# Preparing Overseas Nurses to Work in Australia

## Lee Huang Chiu & Meng Lim

*Drs. Chiu and Lim are the author team for this chapter. They are from the School of Nursing and Midwifery at Victoria University, in Victoria Australia. On its website VU describes itself as a place where "challenging conventional thinking is not only encouraged, it's expected." Drs. Chiu and Lim are fine examples of faculty who focus on improving students' thinking skills to help them challenge conventional wisdom.*

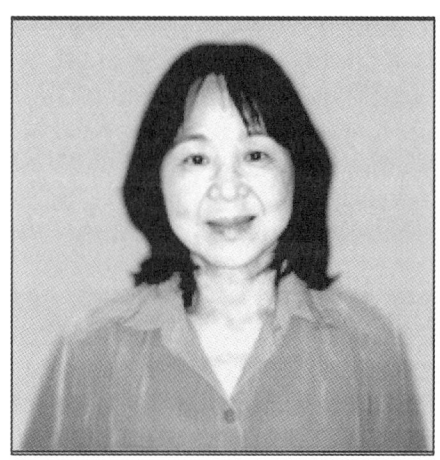

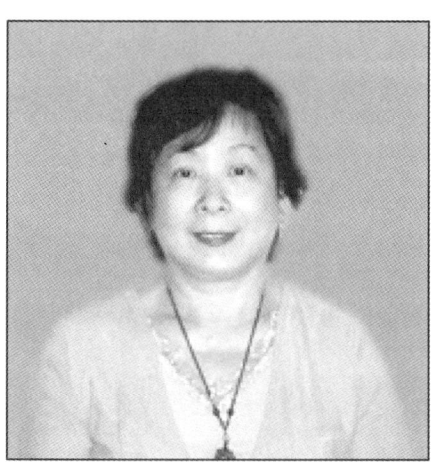

*Dr Lee Huang Chiu [left] is the coordinator of a post graduate course in Orthopedic Nursing, Dr. Meng Lim [above] co-ordinates coursework for overseas qualified and re-entry nurses preparing for their qualification to practice nursing in Australia. Her teaching specialty is postgraduate Pediatric Nursing. Together Drs. Chiu and Lim are committed to helping practicing clinicians appreciate the cultural aspects of care delivery.*

### Class session and students

This lesson uses a case study approach to engage participants to think critically about the influence of ethics, law, and culture. This example lesson is from a class we teach to overseas qualified nurses enrolled in the pre-registration course in the School of Nursing. The majority of these nurses come from Asia and India with a few also coming from Europe. They come to the course with different levels of preparation and experience ranging from a hospital trained certificate to a Diploma of Nursing, with only a few holding the Bachelors Degree in Nursing. Their work experience typically ranges from two to ten years. The pre-registration course is an accredited course which enables overseas qualified nurses to be registered with the Nurses Board of Victoria, Australia. One aim of the course is to familiarize nurses who have been trained overseas with the law and the cultural norms of Australia. We couple this content with readings in ethics and civic policy to prepare these nurses to work competently in Australian health care settings. Another aim is to enable these nurses to register professionally as Division 1 nurses with the Nurses Board of Victoria. The critical thinking skills we emphasize most in the exercise below are interpretation, analysis and explanation .

**The goal of the class session:**

Our goal is to use critical thinking to develop an understanding and awareness of the legal, ethical, professional and cultural issues related to nursing practice in Australia. Students enrolled in the course are mainly from overseas and some are migrants in Australia.

**Learning objectives**

This case study presentation is invaluable in enabling overseas qualified nurses to have the opportunity to use critical thinking to

- Interpret and analyse changing ethical values and the implications of advocacy in nursing;
- Analyse and explain legal issues related to nursing practice;
- Examine the implications of individual and professional accountability with reference to regulation of the profession;
- Analyse and explain the role of culture in providing nursing care within a multicultural society.
- 

**What we do to prepare for this class**

Anticipating the need to discuss important and current issues in practice, we prepare by networking with friends and colleagues who are health care providers in relevant clinical settings to get ideas from them about the most current issues that are raising ethical dilemmas in their workplaces. Once we have identified the issues that will be the focus of the lesson, we conduct a literature search to get updated published information that can inform the class discussion. These relevant reading materials are prepared and handed out to students so that they will come to class ready to think well about the case study dilemmas. Figure 1 is an excerpt from the guidelines for professional and ethical nursing practice in Victoria, Australia. This is an example of the type of material we make available to students for this class session. Here they see evidence that the Australian Board of Nursing has explicit guidelines about being concerned not to coerce patients into compliance and being mindful of a potential abuse of power by the nurse. This is one issue that has relevance to our example case scenario below.

---

**Professional Boundaries**

**Guidelines for Registered Nurses in Victoria**

**4. Principles of safe practice**

- The priority of registered nurses must be to meet the therapeutic needs of their patients.

- In the therapeutic relationship registered nurses need to be aware of their own needs, values and attitudes.

- Registered nurses are responsible for ensuring that the nursing care that they provide is never compromised by putting their own needs ahead of those of their patients.

- Nursing care must never be withheld from a patient as a punishment. Any intent to cause pain or suffering as punishment based on punitive judgement is unacceptable.

- Coercing patient compliance may be an abuse of the power imbalance.

- Registered nurses need to be aware that individual sensitivities, for example cultural differences, may surround some areas of the body when it comes to therapeutic touch, and that these sensitivities are relevant to registered nurses and patients.

---

Figure 1: An excerpt of practice guidelines. NBV: PC – 24 October 2007 Guidelines: Professional Boundaries

## Teaching the lesson

The theory session for this lesson incorporates three main themes: legal issues, ethics and professional practice issues. Case scenarios are used to address the three main themes and to develop students to understand how these themes are relevant to providing nursing care within the Australian Health Care System. The task in this class asks students to apply information about Australian law and the Australian Health Care System to the case scenarios they encounter in the class. As a result they must come to this lesson with some mastery of that material and must have read the readings assigned for the lesson. We've listed some example readings for this class at the end of this chapter.

The learning activity in this lesson requires students to interpret a case study scenario, analyse the patients' health care needs and develop a plan of intervention for the patient. Then the groups are expected to present their analysis of a case study to the class and explain their clinical judgments made on behalf of the patient. We expect students to work in groups of not more than 3 students to undertake this task and to prepare the case study presentation. Each group begins with one of our prepared case studies. Actually we allow then to choose one of the case studies, but each group must present a different case to the class. While they are working, we circle through the groups observing the thinking process being carried on by the group. When it's appropriate and when it does not disturb the process at hand, we point out examples of strong reasoning or interject a question designed to move the group along in their analysis of the case or in their judgment of what could be done for the patient in the case. Here is an actual example of a case study assignment for presentation that is given to students undertaking the class (See Figure 2 below).

**Student Work Product**

We have developed this lesson to include two work products, the group presentation and a written summary of the groups thinking process and clinical judgment. The group presentation should take 45 to 50 minutes and include the opportunity for questions or comments from others in the class. It is expected that students' presentation will demonstrate their ability to utilise the following processes: analysis, synthesis, clinical reasoning, decision-making, group functioning and maintenance, and problem solving. The group case study presentation is the work product for this class exercise. In a course where we use this learning strategy in several class sessions, we can ask a different group to present at each class session. Making the designation of which group will present at the end of the group work time helps each group to work at coming to closure on their possible presentation.

Additionally, a set of presentation criteria are used to assess the groups' ability to think critically about the dilemma of ethical issues that required problem solving to resolve issues that may impact on the value or moral of patient's life. We've included a list of these criteria in Figure 3.

---

Chin Tan is an elderly Chinese man with ischemic foot ulcers and gangrenous toes. The health care team has decided that Chin Tan needs a below knee amputation. He speaks very little English and lives with his daughter. When members of the health care team have tried to talk with him about this, he appears to be slightly confused. He keeps on telling his daughter that he does not want to have his leg cut off. The doctors plan to do the amputation in 2 days time, saying that Chin Tan's daughter has told them her father is aware of the operation and does agree to have it. However, all Chin Tan says to the nursing staff is "Foot no good, foot no good".

Explore the ethics of this case In your small group and prepare a presentation outlining your clinical judgment about how to proceed with this patient dilemma.

The following are some prompts that may assist you to facilitate your discussion:

(1) Read, think and identify: What are the ethical issues in this case study?

(2) Write down: a clear statement about the ethical issues in this case.

(3) Analyse and explain: Which is/are the most central ethical issue(s)? Why?

(4) Analyse, infer and propose: possible explanations for why the issues arose.

(5) Analyse and infer: What evidence is needed to support or disconfirm your explanations for why the ethical issues arose?

(6) Analyse: What possible resources can be used to gather this evidence?

(7) Organise: a plan to access these resources.

(8) Plan how the evidence will be used to make a judgement about how to proceed in the case.

---

**Figure 2: Case Study Scenario Group Task**

The written summary is a submitted overview of the groups' planned case study presentation, including a summary of the major issues evident in the case study. We explain that in this summary the focus should be on demonstrating the critical thinking process that was carried out in the group. We evaluate these summaries by looking for evidence of many of the themes implicit in Figure 2. The written assignment should be brief (about 500 words) and academically written and referenced. Writing brief case summations is an important skill that is also practiced in this exercise, and we look for a concise and organized summary of their presentations written with academic quality in writing skill.

---

All students will be assessed on their ability to:

- Provide a brief preview of the presentation, informing audience about information to be presented
- Provide an adequate rationale for addressing the issue to be discussed
- Communicate information coherently and concisely
- Demonstrate adequate research into the issue by presenting literature search/ review and critical analysis of the literature
- Respond to questions or criticisms from the audience
- Provide a concise summary of major themes
- Provide recommendations for the case where appropriate
- Demonstrate collaborative participation as a group

---

**Figure 3: Criteria for assessing the case presentation**

## One final comment and students' feedback

This exercise is an important one as it engages our students in critical thinking about their understanding and awareness of the legal, ethical, professional and cultural issues that are essential to professional nursing practice in Australia. Students enjoy this learning activity and find it challenging. They have said that it enables them to gain a better understanding of the nursing profession, Australian legal and Health Care Systems, and the related issues implicating nursing practice; and it sharpens their critical thinking skills when they have to read and discern information to solve the problem.

## Recommended Readings

Nurses Act 1993, No 111. (1993). Victorian Government Printing Office (incorporating amendments as of 2000) (Available at http://www.nbv.org.au )
Nurses Board of Victoria (1999). Professional conduct information for registered nurses. Melbourne: Author. (Available at http://www.nbv.org.au )
Nurses Board of Victoria (2001). Professional boundaries. Guidelines for registered nurses in Victoria. Melbourne: Author. (Available at http://www.nbv.org.au )

## Australian Government Legislation used for the class session

(Note: students are not expected to obtain copies of these Acts but are expected to access them as needed)

- Mental Health Act 1986 (Vic)
- Human Tissue Act 1982 (Vic)
- Age of Majority Act 1982 (Vic)
- Medical Treatment Act 1988 (Vic)
- Guardianship and Administration Act 1986 (Vic)
- Mental Health (Amendment) Act 1995
- Health Services Act 1988 (Vic)
- Freedom of information Act 1982 (Vic)
- Privacy Act 2000 (Cth) (available at http://www.privacy.gov.au/act)
- Public Record Act 1973 (Vic)
- Drugs, Poisons & Controlled Substances Act 1981 (Vic)
- Drugs, Poisons & Controlled Substances Regulations 1995 (Vic)
- Nurses Act 1993
- Coroners Act 1985
- Child and Young Persons Act 1989 (Vic)
- Health Professions Registration Act 2005

# Thinking Critically About the Care of Patients with Neurological Disorders

## Kyung Rim Shin

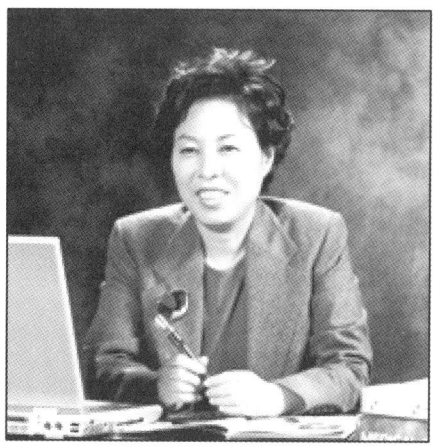

*Dr Kyung Rim Shin is Dean and Professor in the College of Health Science, Ewha Womans University in Seoul, South Korea. She has held many prestigious positions in the discipline of nursing in South Korea, among them the Vice-president of the Korean Nurses Association, the President of the Korean Accreditation Board of Nursing, and the Director of the Korea Center for Qualitative Methodology.*

*We are honored to present Dean Shin's discussion of a class she teaches in the content area of neurological disorders. The use of critical thinking to engage and resolve problems is a habit of mind that requires practice in reflective thinking. Dean Shin's strategy of beginning a class like this with meditative music seems to be an excellent focusing device to impress on students the idea that critical thinking requires the development of good habits of mind. One needs to take the time available to think well, and then find a few moments to subject ones important judgments to the discipline of a fair-minded self critique.*

*There are several very helpful examples in this chapter, but Dean Shin's description of her preparation for this class is of particular value. One can see in her preparation an example of high critical thinking disposition as well as skill. She brings true cases to the classroom, carrying out her own critical thinking exercise in the preparation of those cases. All are informed by the retrieval of actual published research from science journals and national public health reports. This is a method for bringing energy and excellence to the classroom.*

## Class session and students

This class session describes a series of strategies that provide students opportunities to practice their critical thinking skills by applying a portion of course content to a clinical case scenario. I use these strategies often and they would fit well as a progressive introductory thinking exercise and as a practical application of solving clinical problems within any baccalaureate level health science course. In this case the class is about the care of patients with neurological diseases. I usually teach this particular lesson to students who are seniors in an undergraduate nursing program.

**The goal of the class session**

My overall goal in this class is to help students to think critically when they provide nursing care to patients with neurological system problems. I also strive to help them to learn ways of solving problems more independently, managing patient's health problems to arrive at well made clinical judgments about what is needed for the patient.

**Actual materials used for the class session**

I currently assign readings from several current textbooks on medical-surgical nursing and recommend a number of articles for the students to read, three of which are included at the end of the chapter. I also use the current incidence and mortality data for the rates of neurological disorders as they are reported by the Korean National Statistical Office. Most nations post their incidence and mortality data on the Internet now and the statistics for South Korea can be found at the following website: www.kosis.kr. I also use case scenarios of patients with neurological diseases to indicate nursing problems and related care plans. There are also reading requirements for this lesson that include textbooks, selected journal articles, and relevant references that cover the neurological content needed to participate in the class.

**Learning objectives:**

My three main learning objectives for this course are listed below along with mention of the critical thinking skills being strengthen by achieving each of them.

> On completion of this course, the student will be able to:
> - Incorporate assessment of functional health patterns and risk factors into the health history and physical assessment of the patient with neurological conditions. (Interpretation, analysis and inference)
> - Identify the clinical significance and related nursing implications of various tests and procedures used for diagnostic assessment of neurological disorders. (Analysis and explanation)
> - Use the nursing process as a framework of patient care with neurological diseases to:

- o Integrate collected data to derive nursing diagnoses (Inference)
- o Design nursing plans based on nursing diagnoses and evaluate outcomes and the whole process. (Explanation and Evaluation)

**What I do before class**

The case scenarios that will be used by students in the class need to be prepared by me prior to class. Usually, each scenario has two parts, and I distribute Part 1 in the first class hour and Part 2 in the next class hour. This allows me to extend the case with new information and to guide students to reformulate their thinking about the case in light of new information. Figures 1 and 2 display an example of a two part case I've prepared.

To assure that the cases are truly representative of clinical case work, I visit a hospital neurology unit and collect authentic case information that will be relevant to the class content. Using this material, I develop enough case scenarios to provide a unique scenario to each student group. Students also have available the current journal articles and the newest statistical information regarding morbidity and mortality for the neurological disorders represented in the cases. And *then* I prepare my lecture, being sure that I include what will be needed by students to fully address the case scenarios during the class discussion.

For those unfamiliar with these medications, nifedifine it is a calcium channel blocker and mannitol is an osmotic diuretic. Hartmann's solution contains sodium chloride, sodium lactate, and phosphates of calcium and potassium and is used intravenously as a systemic alkalizer and as a fluid and electrolyte replenisher. It is very similar to lactated Ringer's solution an isotonic fluid replacement. This is some of what I am expecting the students to review and evaluate as a part of the case scenario exercise.

The Patient: "A female admitted due to severe headache and general weakness "

A 60year-old female came to Emergency Room because of sudden headache, confusion and general weakness and was transferred to Intensive Care Unit yesterday. She had discontinued her diabetes and hypertension treatment before the symptoms began to occur.

Her orders in the Intensive Care Unit included:

- 5 Liters per minute of oxygen via mask.
- NPO (no food or liquid by mouth)
- Foley catheter
- Fluid monitoring

Today, she is showing a sudden increase in secretions and has developed a stuporous mental state with general edema and facial redness. Her Glasgow Coma Scale score was rated as 11: opened her eyes to pain, used inappropriate words and recoiled to stimulation. Her left pupil is dilated and constricts sluggishly with light stimulation. She also shows an abnormal doll's eye test result. She remains NPO and her fluid balance and electrolyte levels are within normal range. There is no problem with the functioning of her foley catheter.

**Vital Signs:**

- Blood Pressure:     150/100 mm. Hg.
- Heart Rate:         130 beats per minute
- Respiration:        32 breaths per minute
- Temperature:        37.2 degrees Centigrade

FIGURE 1: A CASE SCENARIO SAMPLE

---

The patient has returned from undergoing a Computed Tomography (CT) scan of her brain. Her results show bleeding in the area of the right basal ganglia.

Assessment data collected:

- Vital Signs,
- Glasgow Coma Score,
- pupil size and reflexivity, other brainstem signs

Laboratory studies:

Arterial Blood Gases, a Complete Blood Count (CBC) and blood chemistry were drawn and tested.

Current intravenous medications:

- nifedifine, 25%
- mannitol 50cc x 6
- Hartmann's solution 1000cc

She is remains NPO and with restricted fluids

Urine production remains satisfactory with a functioning foley catheter.

---

**Figure 2: Continuing the Case Scenario**


## How I Teach these Lessons

Before starting the class discussion, I play meditative music to help students relax and to help them to cultivate their thinking ability. I also ask students to group themselves into small working groups for the purpose of working through the class exercise. This offers the same learning environment as clinical practice groups. This lesson in taught in three sections as follows: concept mapping, structured lecture, and discussion of a case scenario. The expectation is that all of the students will have read the assigned reading materials in the textbook and that that will have completed a concept mapping.

***Concept mapping*** is a strategy that requires students to analyze the material that they have read and draw inferences as to the relationships between important key concepts. Students master this skill in previous course work and they apply it here to the topic area of the care of patients with neurological disorders. There are a number of good resources for the use of concept mapping and I've included some of them at the end of the chapter.

During the first hour of this class, each student shares their concept map with the others in a small group discussion, examining and comparing their concept mapping to that drawn by the others. Their task is to refine the varying individual mappings into one complete new concept mapping model. This is a critical thinking exercise that also results in the students synthesizing the knowledge that they have already gained from the readings and the group discussion and also identifying any still needed but unknown knowledge required to master the material.

*Lecture:* The second hour of the class is in lecture format, and I provide a presentation of the information that is in the text, emphasizing all of the knowledge that students need to know. Students can ask any unresolved questions that arose during the concept mapping exercise. Reinforcing the results of a higher order

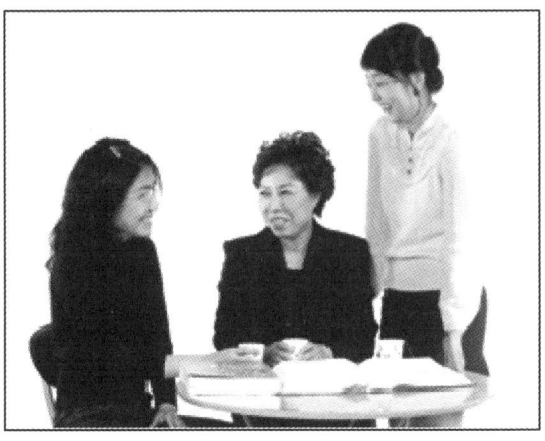

thinking task by providing feedback on the work is an important strategy for teaching the adult learner. Here I present the lecture material after students have worked to organize this new knowledge in the concept mapping. This has the effect of reinforcing students in their use of critical thinking when they have successfully synthesized the content in the concept mapping exercise.

*Case Discussion:* The third hour of class is a discussion of a case scenario that is appropriate for group discussion and is in accordance with the class content. Students synthesize the first two hours of the class lesson by applying this newly gained knowledge to carry out an assessment of the patient in the case scenario I give a different case scenario to each small group (six to seven students) and ask them to work through the case with the following considerations:

- What are the significant cues in the case? Why are they significant?
  (cue recognition- analysis, explanation and inference)
- What is the problem being presented by your patient? What evidence/data grounds this judgment? (hypothesis generation and evidence based clinical judgment– inference and explanation)
- What do you need to discover about the patient or learn about these possible neurological conditions?
  (learning issues: analysis and inference)

These questions are framed to guide the thinking process as student make their clinical judgments about the possible or actual significance of the patients' presenting signs and symptoms and the results of clinical tests. Through the group discussion, students critically decide what health problem is being presented and the possible solutions for addressing that problem. In the course of the discussion they consider functional health patterns and risk factors applicable to the patient using their knowledge of these conditions gained in the earlier part of the class session. They analyze and establish what is known from the health history and the physical assessment of the patient with these neurological conditions. The students arrive at nursing diagnoses and infer priorities using well informed rationale.

I explain to the students that in the actual clinical setting the time allotted for this section of the class would be more than the time available for the care of the scenario patient. But to be sure that this task can be completed in the time available, I ask students to assign learning issues to each group member and then present and share their group's thinking process and findings in the last part of the class session.

**Student Work Product**

I expect that while participating in this type of class, students will analyze any lack of knowledge that they may have in this content area. This is usually well achieved during the individual and group concept mapping exercise. Students also stimulate learning in their peers, can evaluate each others knowledge of neurological disorders, and improve their skills in small group discussion. I evaluate the work that the students do in this class by listening to them use the literature resources and provided epidemiological data to develop a tailored nursing intervention for the scenario patients. They demonstrate their use of critical thinking when they correctly infer social, economic, psychological, and emotional aspects of the case and when they apply an appropriate nursing intervention to the scenarios. In this way, students ultimately can decrease the gap between nursing theory and practice when they apply what they have learned in their future clinic experiences.

Through success in mastering the technique of concept mapping, I expect that students will be better able to synthesize and apply relevant scientific literature as well as grow in their critical thinking self-confidence. Moreover, throughout the analysis of clinical case scenarios in class, students should predictably decrease their fear when they face these same neurological disorders in the real clinical setting and understand better how to address significant health problems in this specialty area.

## Feedback from the students

Students enjoy the opportunity to read and synthesize varying information and epidemiological data when learning about new neurological disorders. They have said that these class exercises help them feel more certain that they understand how to approach patients with signs and symptoms when they can refer to a number of resources to find out more about the disorder than is presented in a single text. Also, they describe the class exercises as stimulating their thinking process in more critical and analytical ways. They also appreciate the opportunity to gain skills in group discussion and plan to use these as possible in hospitals or health care workplaces to carry out nursing strategies for patient care. .

## References

Arbour, R. (2004). Intracranial hypertension: Monitoring and nursing assessment. *Critical Care Nurse*, 24 (5), 19-34.

Carpenito-Moyet, L. *The Understanding the Nursing Process: Concept Mapping and Care Planning for Students*. Philadelphia, PA: Lippincott Williams & Wilkins, 2005.

Evans, R.W. & Olesen, J. (2003). Migraine classification, diagnostic criteria, and testing. *American Academy of Neurology*, 60(7), Supplement 2, S24-S30.

Jennet, B. & Teasdale, G. (1977). Aspects of coma after severe had injury. *The Lancet,* 8107, 878-881.

Kane, M., & Trochim, W. *Concept Mapping for Planning and Evaluation.* Thousand Oaks, CA: Sage Publications, 2006.

Kim, J. (2003). How do U respond to autonomic dysreflexia? *Nursing*, 33 (2), 18.

Moore, L., Lavoie, A., Camden, S., Le Sage, N., Sampalos, J., Bergeron, E., & Abdous, B. (2006). Statistical validation of the Glasgow Coma Score, Journal of Trauma-Injury Infection and *Critical Care,* 60(6), 1238-1244.

Schuster, P. M. *Concept Mapping: A Critical-Thinking Approach to Care Planning.* Philadelphia, PA: F.A. Davis Company, 2002.

# Using the Creative Arts to Develop Critical Thinking Skills: Examining the Qualitative Method of Ethnography

## Beth P. Velde

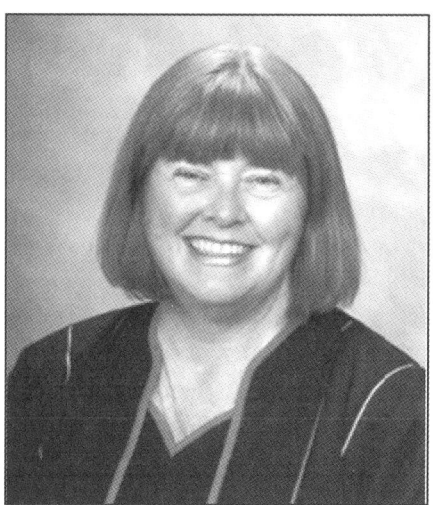

*Dr. Beth Velde is a Professor in Occupational Therapy and an Assistant Dean in the College of Allied Health Sciences at East Carolina University, in Greenville North Carolina, United States. Some of you may have met her in Canada during her doctoral study days at the University of Calgary. Dr. Velde has chaired the Mental Health Association of Pitt County and served on her university's committee on the Status of Women.*

*In this mini-chapter she translates the thinking processes she has learned to do when painting watercolors to help her health sciences students develop their critical thinking skills. This lesson is highly creative and yet it calls for the critical thinking skills of analysis, inference, explanation and evaluation. We particularly like this technique for its ability to expose biases behind our clinical judgments in a way that might be more easily remembered because of the visual depiction and might perhaps be more easily transferred to other analysis and critique contexts.*

## Background

The use of creative arts as a tool in teaching and practicing critical thinking provides an alternative to more traditional discussion or written exercises. Creative artists use critical thinking when they paint. Eight years ago, after taking watercolor lessons, I found that the challenge of completing a painting well required the use of many of the critical thinking skills I was trying to develop in my students. For example, I had to analyze my ideas or concepts to develop a painting, I had to interpret the significant parts of the painting and use them to convey my meaning in the painting to others. This caused me to explore other creative arts for use with my students. I began asking my students to practice their critical thinking skills by painting and drawing.

## Class Session and Students

The creative arts activities described below fit well into many courses and while I use the activities with graduate students, I believe undergraduate students in any of the health sciences could benefit from this type of exercise. Although I usually lead this session, I work as part of a team of four instructors from four different professions (occupational therapy, social work, nursing and health education) and we typically have students from three of these health science professions in the course at any one time. The course is taught as a seminar where the faculty model analytical discussion of the material. There is no specialty knowledge required of the students other than that which is provided in ahead of time the reading material for the class session. It helps if the students are familiar and comfortable with self-reflection. I am presenting the activities for this mini chapter in the context of a qualitative research analysis course that is inter-professional in nature. The specific example in this lesson is a class where ethnography is the method being discussed.

## The goal of the class session

This class session introduces ethnography as a way of analyzing ideas and so one clear goal of the course is that students will increase their ability to see the influence of culture on interpersonal interactions. I help them to do this through their critical reflection on the readings assigned for the course, and particularly the session at hand, and through their portrayal of the lesson content through three creative arts activities. They interpret, analyze draw inferences about, and evaluate the material (critical thinking skills in action). I want them to develop these skills so they can better develop research proposals and conduct qualitative research. I believe the activity of viewing and discussing another student's creative activities also fosters the critical thinking skills of analysis and inference.

## The material used for the class session

Students are asked to read a chapter on ethnography and also an assigned research article that provides an example of this research methodology. Any excellent text on qualitative research that clearly communicates the method in question will serve equally well to provide the methods content. In many cases one would want to find an example of excellent research design. But for this lesson that involves critique, I have found that more is learned if the published study that I assign states it is "ethnography" (or phenomenology, grounded theory, etc) but demonstrates methods or results that somehow do not conform to the principles of research design that is described in the book. In this case I will be expecting the students to identify the methodological weaknesses in the published article. This conflict promotes questioning and helps students feel more comfortable in critiquing published research.

I also spend a bit of time before class thinking about specific questions that I might ask during the discussions. The classroom environment is critical to the success of this activity. I arrive at the room early so I can set up the tables in a rectangle and leave an open area for the statues activity. I have blank paper and pencils for the drawing activity.

## Learning Objectives

Students will be able to:

1. Accurately evaluate the research article using the criteria for good ethnographic research described in the text.
2. Interpret for their classmates the concepts of quality for good ethnographic research using a creative arts activity.
3. Defend their portrayal to their peers and verbally justify their interpretation of the ideas presented in the text.
4. Examine their own biases about qualitative research and make them observable using a creative arts activity.

## How I Teach this Lesson

The week before this session, I remind students to critically read the article and the book chapter. By this, I mean that they should be attentive to interpreting what is being communicated in the chapter and article, and carefully analyze, evaluate and compare any claims being made by the authors of each reading. I suggest they record "jottings" of their ideas on a piece of paper and I talk about the concept of jotting versus taking narrative notes, underlining or highlighting.
I explain that jottings are ways to remember the essence of the information in the reading—not complete sentences and not extracting quotes from the reading. They are a way for the student to remember the reading and are often done in a type of shorthand, using abbreviations and even symbols.

I open the seminar by asking each student to draw a picture of what their inner self looks like as they reflect on the chapter content. They can use the jottings about the chapter as a reflective tool. I ask them not to talk, but to work silently and thoughtfully. I also tell them it is ok to use stick figures and to draw the picture like a cartoon. The cartoon may convey humor, may be satirical, or may be serious in nature. It tells a story and is meant to evoke an emotional response. Sometimes I tell them to draw the first two frames of a four-frame cartoon. The first two frames are drawn based on their original perspective on the reading and the last two on their perspective after we have discussed the reading in class.

In the course of creating the drawing, I want my students to examine their feelings about the material. I am hoping that they will assess their confidence in their own interpretation of the material, and be honest about what they feel they know and don't know. Faculty also do this activity and they share their drawings as well. This is important because many students respond to the activity by saying "I can't draw". They need to see that faculty also struggle with creative activities and that the purpose here is not to be an artist, but to identify each person's interpretation and analysis of the text and examine the accuracy of the interpretations. This activity takes 10 minutes.

After the drawings are complete, I and my colleague faculty ask each student to pass his or her drawing to the student sitting next to them and to talk about the drawing. After they discuss their drawing, the other student (the reviewer) writes comments underneath the drawing. The comments are meant to clarify any questions that were identified in the discussion of the drawing.

- What the main idea/point of…?
- How does ….effect/influence the outcome?
- What if …happened?
- How does that relate to ….?
- Can you explain why….?"
- What conclusions can you draw about…?
- What is the difference between…and…?
- How are….and….similar?
- How would I use….to….?
- What is the best...and why?"

**Figure 1: Question frames that put the emphasis on critical thinking**

The next step is to share the drawings with the class. The class itself is set up as a seminar and the tables and chairs form a large square. Typically a faculty member sets the stage by sharing their drawing first, unless a student is comfortable beginning. As faculty, our job is asking questions that will promote higher level thinking skills. As a guide, I use King's (1991) guided reciprocal peer questioning technique. Examples of question frames that work in this activity are shown in Figure 1.

As faculty, I intentionally model the use of these questions. In addition, at the beginning of the course I talk about the use of questioning and the patterns of interaction in a graduate level class. I intentionally reward interaction between students and try to redirect interaction and questions posed to faculty by students. Often times, I answer a question with a question.

The discussion takes 40 minutes. In the course of this discussion, all of the important content about the research methodology comes into the discussion, offered by the students themselves as it is relevant to their critique of the research article. *There is never a need for didactic presentation of the chapter material.* If they miss anything important about the critique of the study, one of the faculty can add these comments.

After I use the drawings as a focus for the chapter analysis, I ask students and faculty to review their jottings on the methodology, as well as the results and the discussion of the research article. Then I ask them to work in groups of three to create a statue that portrays a part of the research article. There are two variations I have used in this respect. If I have chosen a study for the seminar where the methodology of the study violates the principles of ethnography (contradicts the book chapter's description of ethnography), then I ask them to create a statue about the method actually used in the article. If the study's results do not represent the outcomes of ethnography, then I ask them to portray the results. In this case, one person is the sculptor and two are the "clay." Again, the faculty participate in the entire activity as a way of putting students at ease with the creative process. After 3 or 4 minutes, I ask the statue to freeze. I then tap the shoulders of some statue groups and ask them to walk around and view the other statues. They take turns as viewers and statues.

We discuss the statues and each sculptor explains her statue. We ask the students to explain why they believe the study does not conform to the concepts in the book, and each group provides their analysis and evaluation of the article as it is depicted in their statue. Sometimes I ask the sculptors to change the statue so that the statue is even more representative of the description of ethnography in the book. This part of the discussion is a particularly important piece because it challenges students to reexamine their interpretation of ethnography and to evaluate their prior critical thinking about the research article. In attempting to change the statue they go a bit deeper with their evaluation of the article based on the book. This activity takes 25 minutes.

Finally, at the end of every class students are required to reflect on the classroom experience. I provided guided activities to build their ability to reflect and the one I use for this class session is to have students write a haiku. Figure 2 displays the directions that are given. This activity takes 15 minutes.

---

Write a haiku. Haiku is a form of poetry through which you express yourself and your impressions of the world. Haiku has a specific meter that is created by a set number of syllables in the poem, Here is one way to create an haiku.

- Begin by naming ethnography in your own words.
- Now, describe it.
- Name a setting where ethnographies occur, and describe the setting.
- Describe the feelings that you have about the image you made about ethnography.
- Now, go back through what you've written and underline the key words and phrases that really describe the essence of ethnographies.
- Move these around and play with them in your mind until there are only 17 syllables: one line of five syllables, one of seven syllables, and another line of five syllables.

---

Figure 2: Haiku exercise

## What I Expect from the Class Participants

All four faculty in our teaching team are strong believers in active learning strategies and all are comfortable challenging each other during class time, modeling the value of peer questioning. Because we take turns each week as the course leader, we collaborate on the types of activities used. I expect all students to participate both verbally and physically in the activities of this session. I modify the physical environment so they are safe, and we close the door so the classroom is private and to lesson their discomfort during the statue activity. Because everyone participates there is less a sense of an audience. The creative activities provide an alternative way to express questions.

This session is part of a course that is available for students at the masters or doctoral level as an elective. There are no examinations, but students complete a portfolio that includes classroom activities, reading and class reflections, a photography project, a research proposal, and a field observation. The portfolio is graded by all four instructors using a rubric that incorporates critical thinking

*Using the Creative Arts to Develop Critical Thinking* 263

cognitive skills that we expect throughout the portfolio. Figures 3 is an example of a drawing from a seminar where the chapter reading as on the topic of 'bracketing' and the research article was (Johnson & Samdahl, 2005).

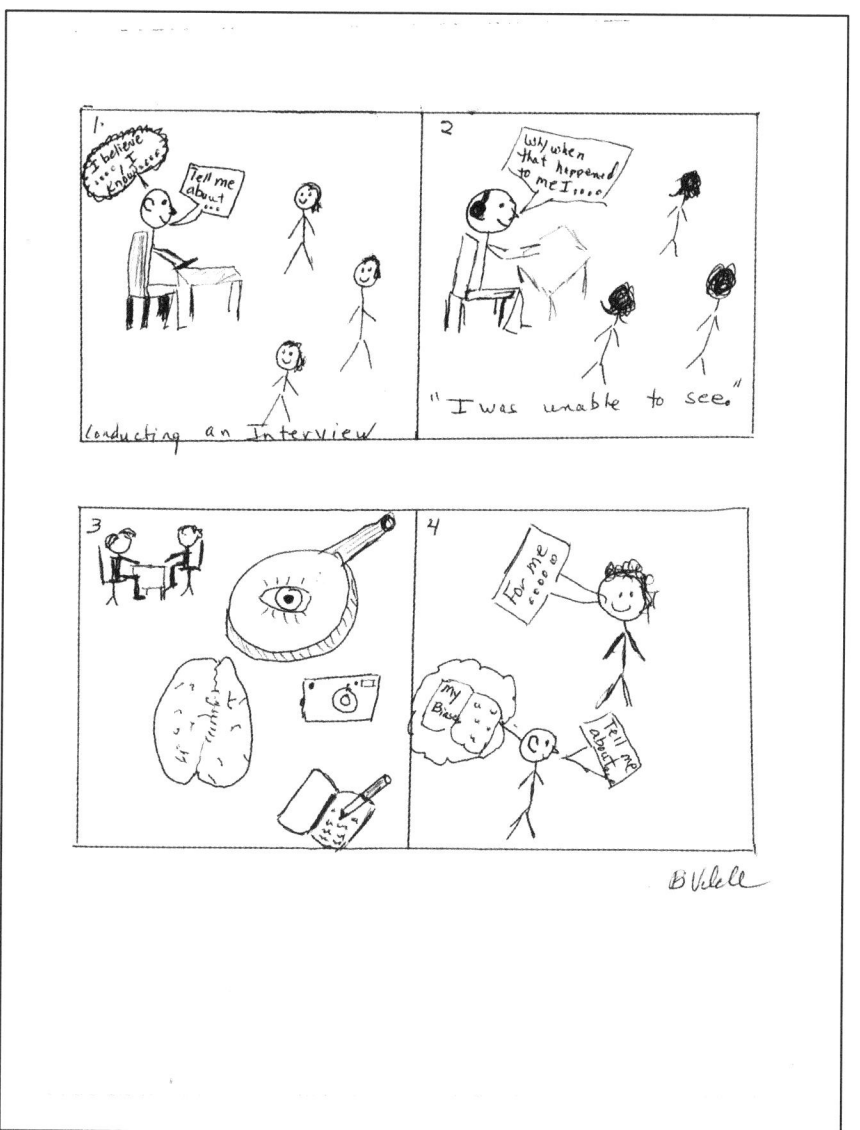

The following is an excerpt of the artist's explanation of her drawing.

"The readings helped me understand that to really hear someone's story I need to identify my own beliefs and my sense of privilege. I think people choose their research topic because it resonates for them in their own way. That makes them especially vulnerable to assuming their research participants will feel and describe experiences in the same way they do. ...They are at risk for ignoring the data....and vulnerable to only seeing similarities in the data. The readings made me think about how I would recognize my biases and assumptions that come from my own culture and realize this type of self-reflection and analysis is very hard. ...My own culture is hidden to me. I had to really think about the differences between a bias and an assumption.

"My drawing shows me the first time I interviewed. I was the one in control so I am seated and everyone else is standing. I dominate the drawing. The others are talking but nothing is coming out of their mouths because I can only hear what is in my head. The cultural elements of a desk and a chair separate me from my participants. The second panel shows what happened to the interview, the others have turned their backs on me, they know I don't want to listen.

"The third panel is my research director talking with me, reflecting my stance and my sense of privilege. I think about what she says, I write about it, I take pictures that represents what I know, I keep a diary. The last panel is me with a research participant again. I am listening, I am standing just like my participant. My culture's symbols of power—the desk, is gone. My participant is the dominant person and I am trying to keep my biases in check."

**Feedback from the Students**

Students comment on two areas. The first is the manner in which the course is conducted, when they see the faculty as active participants, not just the "sage on the stage". On occasion, when faculty disagree with each other, we have had students indicate they don't know "who to believe." As we know our students are still striving to advance their cognitive development, we model respectfully voicing disagreements and potentially conflicting points of view, demonstrating how to assess these opposing arguments. By the end of the course, students identify this as a true strength of the course.

The second area is the emphasis on active learning and critical thinking. While we occasionally post Microsoft PowerPoint™ presentations to call attention to some key areas in readings, our course style is reflected in the description of the session above. Students are required to be interactive and to express their learning using more than one sensory system. Again, by the end of the course students express their appreciation for the holistic manner of presentation and their own efficacy in being researchers.

**Reference**

Johnson, C.W. & Samdahl, D.M. (2005). "The Night *They* Took Over: Misogyny in a Country-Western Gay Bar. *Leisure Sciences, 27*(3), 331-348.

King, A. (1991). Enhancing Peer Interaction and Learning in the Classroom through Reciprocal Questioning. *American Educational Research Journal,* 27, 664-687.

# Working with Patients Who Self-Harm

## Margaret McAllister

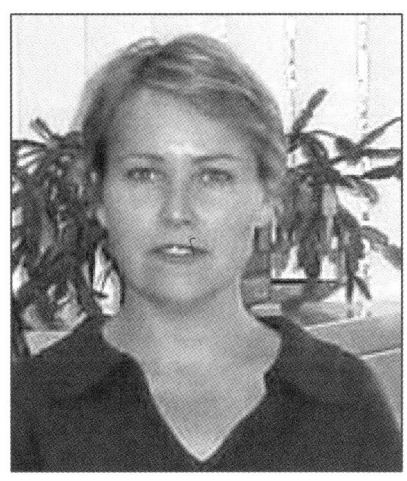

*Dr Margaret McAllister is an Associate Professor in Nursing at the School of Health and Sport Sciences, at the University of the Sunshine Coast in Maroochydore, Queensland, Australia. Previously she was faculty in the School of Nursing and Midwifery at Griffith University in Queensland Australia. Dr. McAllister has a certification in psychiatric nursing and particular expertise in therapeutic responses to self-injury and in critical social theory. She reminds us in this chapter that while students or clinicians will use the full range of critical thinking skills in a practice exercise, some of the best teaching sessions are focused in one skill area.*

*The exercise in this chapter requires students to use the critical thinking skill of analysis, using a rich assortment of teaching methods. Not forgotten are the critical thinking habits of mind that prove so needed for a fair-minded analysis of the problems presenting to patients who self harm. This is a very rich chapter with at least three creative and well integrated reasoning exercises that require students to apply mental health content in a clinical relevant context. The connection between using critical thinking skills and making a well grounded clinical judgment is evident.*

*Dr. McAllister has also authored a book entitled, "Solution Focused Nursing: Rethinking Practice." We took a moment to look in to this text and found a treasure that extends to the web based companion text site which coaches novice teachers or those new to this content area to bring this material to students with care to completely engage them in critical thinking pedagogy.*

## The Session and the Participants

This session is one that I offer to professionals and health science students who are interested in developing their intervention skills when working with individuals who deliberately self-injure. The session participants are typically from a range of disciplinary backgrounds and include: teachers, youth workers, nurses, social workers, psychologists, disability support workers and medical officers.

**The Lesson**

This lesson focuses on the practice of clinical problem solving in the context of working with patients who self-harm. My key goals for the class session involve all of the following:

1. emphasizing the importance of a holistic approach to problem solving

2. increasing awareness of the role that solution searching/generating has for clinicians/clients in the problem solving process

3. emphasizing the importance of a balanced appreciation of clients' vulnerabilities and strengths

4. emphasizing the importance and effects of building a sense of community between clinicians and clients

5. developing skills in working with clients' strengths, aspirations and solutions

My particular focus for this session is to develop the critical thinking skill of *analysis*. Participants have an opportunity to examine how dominant ways to problem-solving are enacted in clinical settings. I help them to do this through participating and debriefing a role play and brainstorm exercise.

The critical thinking dispositions of *systematicity, open-mindedness and truth-seeking* (APA, 1990) are also frequently emphasized as a function of my philosophy of practice and my teaching methods. Finally I try to impress on the participants the value of working with clients to help them problem solve.

This lesson is divided into three main sections: A content loaded slideshow; a role play exercise and a brainstorming exercise. Together they address the following learning outcomes.

## The Learning Objectives

Clinicians and other professionals who participate in this session will be able to:

- Critically analyze the dominant ways in which the problem solving process has been used in health services and the impact this can have on patients who self-injure.

- Describe the need for a balanced perspective on clients' vulnerabilities and strengths. (open-mindedness and truth-seeking) and use this perspective to analyze and draw accurate inferences about a client's vulnerabilities and strengths, problem identification and solution generation. (analysis, inference).

- Describe the benefits of living in a close community and explain the importance building a sense of community between clinicians and clients (analysis, explanation).

## How I teach the lesson

***The slide show:*** Thinking well about a problem requires best knowledge of the problem in context so I begin the less with a slide show that provides needed content. The slide show also introduces about problem solving and solution searching as well as content about the etiology and incidence of self harming behavior. Figure 1 is an example slide from that presentation. My slides are visual aids accompanying a short talk on what is known about the problem of patients who self harm. While the participants view the slides I explain why the problem is so important and that we think we know about intervening.

Here is some of what I tell them (references for this material are included at the end of this chapter). Self-injurers represent nearly one percent of the population, with a higher proportion of females than males. The typical onset of self-harming acts is at puberty. The behaviours often last for five to ten years but can persist much longer without appropriate treatment. It is impossible to know the exact prevalence of self-injury because there is no clear, simple definition, and the act is usually done in secret. We can, however, get an idea of the prevalence from hospital separations, where self-harm occurs in 4% of the Australian population, as well as samples of Australian secondary school students where the prevalence of self-injury has been recorded as 5.1%, 6.2%, and 10.5%.International figures are similar to Australian trends (Berry & Harrison, 2006).

People who self-injure place considerable burden on health care systems. In 1999 suicide and self-inflicted injuries represented 27% of the total injury burden in Australia; equal to road traffic accidents. The annual wider economic burden of self harm is estimated at $160 million and the total health costs of injuries is estimated at $2.6 billion (8.3%) of total health expenditure. The World Health Organization has produced information about 'at risk' youth all over the developed world (WHO, 2000). We know they have the following characteristics:

- They live in impoverished, inner city neighbourhoods
- They have many stressors including: prenatal and post natal exposure to drugs, parental depression, abandonment, inconsistent parenting, poverty and hunger, high rates of parental unemployment.
- They exhibit many of all of the following: physical and psychosocial developmental delays, malnutrition, missed schooling, inadequate health care, involvement in crime, drug use, and risky sexual behaviour.

### Young people and self-injury

- Self-injury is a taboo and so statistics are tentative
- Prevalence is 4 % in Australian Populations (AIHW, 2000)
- In Adolescent **inpatient** settings: 40-61% (Kress et al, 2004)
- Higher proportion in **girls** than boys (Stagg, 2005)
- Typical **age** of onset : puberty, and often lasts for 5-10 yrs
- Costly: 27% of injury burden in Australia, equal to MVA
- Annual **economic burden** $160 Million, 8.3% of total health expenditure,
- 5% seen at hospital after self-harm will have **suicide**d within 9 years (Stagg, 2005) At the time though, few involve suicidal in ten t (Nada-Raja et al 2004)
- Many are likely to be discharged **without** a completed psychosocial assessment or follow-up (Bennewith et al, 2005)

Figure 1: Example content slide for Slide presentation

**Small Group Role Play Exercise:** To begin this next part of the session, I divide the participants into groups of three persons each. One person in the group will play the role of the 'patient' and I provide them a script to read as they play this role (Figure 2).

---

**The script for the Patient Role**

Please read this script, take a few moments to think about Alice and how she would behave, and then engage in an interview with the clinician as though you were Alice. Take your time during the interview and be thoughtful about your responses to the clinicians questions. Don't reveal any of these things unless you both feel you can trust the clinician and he/she explicitly asks you about the nature and extent of your self-harm.

**SCRIPT**

Your name is Alice. You are 17 years old and you have been brought to the ED by your friends, who were concerned about hearing you vomiting in the bathroom. You have previously been a psychiatric patient, and although you were only 16 you were told you had Borderline Personality Disorder and Bulimia.

You know that you have disordered eating, and are frequently bulimic. But you don't want to stop your purging behavior because you find it helps you cope with your emotional eating. At least it keeps your weight under control. You also self-harm – you've cut your wrists many times. You do this because sometimes you feel zoned out, not real. When you cut yourself it makes you feel real again, and at least it shows you that you're alive. You also have a shameful secret – you have recently cut the inside of your thighs but you don't want to tell anyone this. You feel like cutting is part of your identity and you would be afraid to stop.

---

**Figure 2**

Another person in the group plays the 'clinician' who is a member of the psychiatric liaison team. I explain to this person that they have been asked to assess the patient. They have the following materials available to assist this process: some brief triage case notes (Figure3), a Deliberate Self Harm (DSH) Form (Figure 4) and a score on the 'Sadperson's Scale' (Figure 5, Hockberger and Rothstein, 1987). The DSH Form is a pathway form that we have created for our local facility that collects patient intake data on a variety of key variable in order to determine a triage level and risk profile.

> **Triage Case Notes for the Clinician Role**
>
> - Admit: 2300 hours: Patient presented with friends to the Emergency Department
> - Note: Past history as a private psychiatric patient.
> - Diagnosis: Bipolar Disorder (BPD) and Bulimia
> - Name: Alice
> - Age: 17
> - Presenting complaint: teenage friends heard her in the bathroom vomiting. Didn't know what to do or who to contact so they brought her to the Emergency Department.
> - Action: place on category 3 (as not actively suicidal and can wait 20 minutes). For Referral to psychiatric liaison team. Acquire psychiatric chart.

**Figure 3**

> **Deliberate Self Harm (DSH) pathway form**
>
> Intake guideline for the DSH form:
>
> 1. Evidence of self harm (Self injury, overdose, both)
> 2. If medical injury outweighs need for psychiatric assessment institute treatment first: (Record of treatment given)
> 3. Emotional state (conflict, loss, anger, depression)
> 4. Suicide related history and current behavior
> 5. Known psychiatric disease
> 6. Substance abuse
> 7. Current Medication
> 8. Psychosocial assessment (conducted by physician)

**Figure 4**

I tell the clinician that they are to conduct a health assessment using these standard forms and procedures. The third person in the group plays the 'critical friend' to the clinician. I give the critical friend a private message telling that that they are to carry out an appraisal of the practice behavior (patient assessment) of their friend the clinician without forewarning. They are to assess his/her problem solving and solution searching skills by filling out an Evaluation Form (Figure 6) and they will be discussing their feedback with the group.

# Sadpersons Scale

**Note:**

A score of over 6 requires intensive management (which may include hospitalisation).

| | | Description | Score |
|---|---|---|---|
| **S** | Sex | Male | 1 |
| **A** | Age | If <19 or >45 | 1 |
| **D** | Depression or hopelessness | Admits to depression or decreased concentration, appetite, sleep, libido | 2 |
| **P** | Previous attempts or psychiatric care | Previous in patient or outpatient psychiatric care | 1 |
| **E** | Excessive alcohol or drug use | Stigmata of chronic addiction or recent frequent use | 1 |
| **R** | Rational thinking loss | Organic brain syndrome or psychosis | 2 |
| **S** | Separated, divorced or widowed | | 1 |
| **O** | Organised or serious attempt | Well thought out plan, or "life threatening" presentation | 2 |
| **N** | No social supports | No close family, friends, job or active religious affiliation | 1 |
| **S** | Stated future intent | Determined to repeat attempt or ambivalent | 2 |

Reprinted from Publication: *The Journal of Emergency Medicine*, Vol. 6, Hockberg, R. & Rothstein, R. "Assessment of Suicide Potential by Non-Psychiatrists Using the SAD PERSON score," pp. 99-107. (1987), with permission from Elsevier.

Figure 5

## Assessing the Clinician's Response to the Case Study Role Play

Rate the quality of the clinical interaction using the criteria specified. It's important that you be fair-minded and honest with this evaluation. Be prepared to provide examples for your ratings. (Ask yourself: Why do I think that this interaction was exemplary/adequate/limited/inadequate?)

| Criteria | Degree of Understanding and Clinical Judgment | | | | | |
|---|---|---|---|---|---|---|
| | Exemplary | Adequate response | Limited but safe response | Limited and potentially inadequate response | Inadequate response | N/A |
| Engaging attributes are apparent | | | | | | |
| Concerns and issues are considered effectively, safely and thoroughly | | | | | | |
| Self-harm understanding is conveyed appropriately to the person | | | | | | |
| Future coping and resilience are considered | | | | | | |

Describe 3 key strengths (these comments should address more positive ratings)

1 _____

2 _____

3 _____

Describe 3 areas for improvement (these must address all inadequate ratings)

1 _____

2 _____

3 _____

Figure 6: Evaluation Form to be completed by the Critical Friend

In order to debrief students in this roleplay, the class is asked to comment on the experience of asking questions and being asked probing questions. Then they are to find common strengths and areas for improvement in their clinical interactions. This helps to move students beyond the clinical context towards future learning experiences.

If time permits, the roles in the group can be shifted and a new patient script (case study) can be provided. This has the advantage of the group working increasingly toward achieving the criteria being evaluated by the critical friend. But in most cases, unless this is a daylong workshop, you will need to move on to the brainstorming exercise.

***The Brainstorm -- What is a Healthy Community?*** Helping youth to find a healthy community is one way to intervene in the problem of self-harm. This part of the session asks participants to turn their minds to thinking about the notion of community. My comments go something like this: "Before we think about a great community, let's think for a moment about some of the stories in the media that signal to us the *breakdown of community.*" At this point I again use visual aids to help the participants think about examples of community. I show them eight or ten images that could be analyzed in relationship to the concept of community. For example I might show them the following collection of images: a group of students celebrating their graduation, a child holding an infant in a third world country, two dogs standing together in a metal cylinder, a woman sitting on the sidewalk with a request for food printed on a square of cardboard, neighbors working together on a community project. After giving everyone some time to view the images, to analyze what they represent, what feelings they engender, I ask volunteers to select one image and say why it resonated for them. "What meanings did the image hold, and what effects of community or deficiency in community did you interpret in the image?"

When participants are asked to brainstorm about the attributes of the breakdown of community, they typically generate comments like the following: community's lack of care, dehumanising each other, failing to act to help others, caring for the self above others, inhumane treatments... leading to demoralization, devaluing self and others, loss of hope, disregard, apathy, competitiveness, ego-centrism, violence...When asked to brainstorm about a *good community*, or a *healthy community,* their responses typically include phrases like this: every person is known; each has a role and feels valued; there are rituals that are enriching and rewarding; people are helpful, compassionate, and caring; there is a sense of belonging, fun, achievement; there are celebrations; milestones are marked.

Brainstorming isn't always reliable so if they fail to mention something important, I add this material myself. To wrap up of the session, I ask participants to relate their insights to how we might support individuals who self harm in the clinical environment if we were to use some of these features of a healthy community.

**Assessing learning outcomes in a participant work product**

To assess the learning goals students complete the individual work activity. This gives opportunity for students to demonstrate their analytic thinking and creative solution generation skills. It also records evidence of their thinking process (Figure 7).

### Individual Activity
### Building a healthy sense of self and community with patients

Your task is to devise activities that will help you work with an individual client to build their awareness of their personal strengths and the specific goals they would like to achieve. Use this suggested format to organize and present your ideas. Use all that you have learned in this session to provide your rationale for the activities you suggest.

| Feature of a healthy Community | Your activity | Patient's activity | Rationale |
|---|---|---|---|
| People are familiar and known | | | |
| Sense of purpose | | | |
| Sense of belonging | | | |
| Shared places | | | |
| Shared ideas | | | |
| Shared memories | | | |
| Other: | | | |

Figure 7

# References

Auditor General for Western Australia T. *Life Matters: Management of Deliberate Self-Harm in Young People*. Audit. Perth: Western Australian Government; 2001. Report No.11.

Bennewith, O., Peters, T., Hawton, K., House, A., & Gunnell, D. (2005). Factors associated with the non-assessment of self-harm patients attending an Accident and Emergency Department: Results of a national study. *Journal of Affective Disorders,* 89(1-3), 91-97.

Berry, J. & Harrison, J. (2006). *Hospital separations due to injury and poisoning, Australia 2003-04.*' Available on line at http://www.nisu.flinders.edu.au/pubs/reports/2007/injcat88.php the Australian Institute of Health and Welfare

Hockberger, R. & Rothstein, R. (1987). Assessment of suicide potential by nonpsychiatrists using the SAD PERSONS score. *The Journal of Emergency Medicine*, 6(2), 99-107.

House, A., Owens, D., & Patchett, L. (1999). Deliberate self harm. *Quality in Health Care,* 8:137-143.

Kress, V., Gibson, D., & Reynolds, C. (2004). Adolescents who self-injure: Implications and strategies for school counsellors. *American Professional School Counsellors Association Journal, 7* (3), 195-201

McAllister, M. (2003). Multiple meanings of self harm: a critical review. *International Journal of Mental Health Nursing*. 12(3), 177-85.

McAllister, M, Tower, M. & Walker R. (2007). Gentle interruptions: transformative approaches to clinical teaching. *Journal of Nursing Education*, 46(7), 304-12.

McAllister, M. (Ed.) *Solution Focused Nursing; Rethinking Practice*. Houndmills, England, Palgrave Macmillan Publishers, 2007.

Nada-Raja, S., Skegg, K., Langley, J., Morrison, D., & Sowerby, P. (2004). Self-harmful behaviours in a population based sample of young adults. *Suicide and Life Threatening Behavior, 34*, 177-86.

Skegg, K. (2005). Self-harm. *Lancet,* 366: 1471-83.

Steenkamp, M. & Harrison, J. *Suicide and hospitalised self harm in Australia*. Canberra: Australian Institute of Health and Welfare; 2000.

Van der Kolk, B., Perry, C., & Herman J. (1991) Childhood origin of self destructive behaviour. *American Journal of Psychiatry*. 148 (12), 1665-1671.

# Training the Discovery of Evidence of Critical Thinking

## Peter A. Facione

### Background

*Sometimes the best learning experiences come from efforts to teach with a mind toward evaluation. Consideration of how one might measure the achievement of learning goals forces one to develop a clear understanding of what evidence of learning should be observable in the classroom or clinic.*

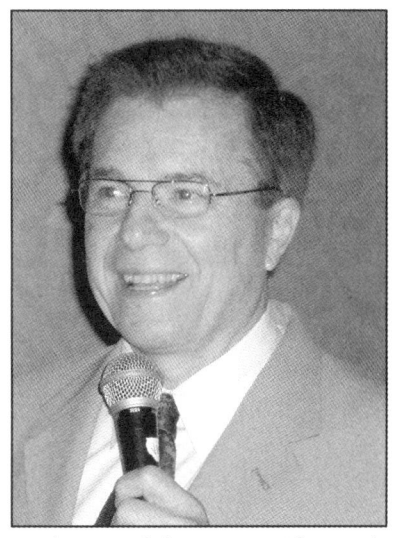

*Noreen and I developed the Holistic Critical Thinking Scoring Rubric (HCTSR) in 1994 in response to requests for a tool which (a) could be used to evaluate a variety of educational work products including essays, presentations, and demonstrations, and (b) works as both a pedagogical device to guide people to know what critical thinking is as well as an assessment tool useful for both formative and summative purposes. The HCTSR, integrates both the skills and the dispositions involved in critical thinking, and is available as a free download from its publisher, The California Academic Press / Insight Assessment www.insightassessment.com/hctsr.html and has been republished in numerous texts on the teaching of critical thinking. We attribute this rubric's wide popularity with educators across many disciplines and professional fields to its ability to describe levels of quality in reasoning using common language. Another rubric we've developed is the Professional Judgment Rating Form (PJRF), intended for use in rating demonstrated critical thinking skills and disposition in simulation labs and clinical placement settings.*

### How I use the HCTSR

One of my favorite lessons with the HCTSR is taught not to students but to experienced faculty colleagues. Typically at a professional conference workshop on learning outcomes assessment I use it in an exercise intended to demonstrate how rubrics are developed and used. But more importantly, I use it as a way of helping faculty to identify evidence of a thinking process embedded in a piece of written work or in an oral presentation. If we are to teach fellow clinicians or health science students how to better approach clinical problems, it is imperative that we train ourselves to be better at hearing the thinking of those we mentor and skilled at helping them to analyze their thinking for its quality. The HCTSR can be used by anyone to rate thinking, but the ratings will be flawed unless the rater can identify evidence of strong or weak critical thinking.

The exercise is also useful for showing the importance of establishing inter-rater reliability as a precondition for the valid and reliable use of rubrics as summative assessment tools. In this case the inter rater reliability rests on the group's ability to identify evidence of strong or weak critical thinking skill or disposition.

The demonstration goes as follows: We read the HCTSR together talking about the construct of "critical thinking" so that we all understand at an abstract level what this tool is intended to measure. We talk about disciplining ourselves to respond to the critical thinking manifested in the student work, and not other important but separate features of that work product, such as its factual correctness, its grammar or its writing quality. Again, while these elements are essential for an overall evaluation of a student's project, at the moment our focus is on the critical thinking involved. Typically everyone in the workshop, experienced faculty one and all, understands the distinctions that need to be made and promises to focus only on the critical thinking when they apply the HCTSR to the actual student work.

That understood, I distribute a small number of short essays written by students on some controversial topic, e.g. genetic modification of foods. Any piece of student work that requires them to discuss a decision making process can be used for this exercise as it could reasonably be expected to contain evidence of the student's thinking process. I use essays that were written spontaneously, meaning that the students did not have the chance to do any preparation or gather any data prior to being asked, in class, to spend 20 minutes writing their opinions and explaining their reasons. The faculty in the workshop are provided with a description of the essay writing assignment and invited to rate the essays using the HCTSR (see below). After a suitable period of time, the great majority have given a score: 4, 3, 2 or 1, to each of the essays. A rating of 3 is a good score, and a 4 is a very good score. Similarly a 2 is a poor score, but 1 is far worse. We then tally the scores for each essay, and inevitably we find that on some essays there is reasonable consensus. For instance, all or most of the

## The Holistic Critical Thinking Scoring Rubric
P. Facione and N. Facione

### 4. Consistently does all or almost all of the following:

Accurately interprets evidence, statements, graphics, questions, etc.
Identifies the salient arguments (reasons and claims) pro and con.
Thoughtfully analyzes and evaluates major alternative points of view.
Draws warranted, judicious, non-fallacious conclusions.
Justifies key results and procedures, explains assumptions and reasons.
Fair-mindedly follows where evidence and reasons lead.

### 3. Does most or many of the following:

Accurately interprets evidence, statements, graphics, questions, etc.
Identifies relevant arguments (reasons and claims) pro and con.
Offers analyses and evaluations of obvious alternative points of view.
Draws warranted, non-fallacious conclusions.
Justifies some results or procedures, explains reasons.
Fair-mindedly follows where evidence and reasons lead.

### 2. Does most or many of the following:

Misinterprets evidence, statements, graphics, questions, etc.
Fails to identify strong, relevant counter-arguments.
Ignores or superficially evaluates obvious alternative points of view.
Draws unwarranted or fallacious conclusions.
Justifies few results or procedures, seldom explains reasons.
Regardless of the evidence or reasons, maintains or defends views
    based on self-interest or preconceptions.

### 1. Consistently does all or almost all of the following:

Offers biased interpretations of evidence, statements, graphics, questions,
    information, or the points of view of others.
Fails to identify or hastily dismisses strong, relevant counter-arguments.
Ignores or superficially evaluates obvious alternative points of view.
Argues using fallacious or irrelevant reasons, and unwarranted claims.
Does not justify results or procedures, nor explain reasons.
Regardless of the evidence or reasons, maintains or defends views
    based on self-interest or preconceptions.
Exhibits close-mindedness or hostility to reason.

faculty have given an essay a positive score (4 or 3) or a negative score (2 or 1). But, and I set it up this way intentionally, there is always at least one essay where the rating is not as obvious and we discover that the group has assigned the full spectrum of scores, with the majority of scores being 3's or 2's.

We then debrief the situation together. Splitting the ratings more or less equally across 'good' and 'poor' scores is not a good situation, obviously. If this had been a "pass-fail" assessment, which rating would it have been? Pass or fail? If the student had been lucky (unlucky) enough to have registered in a section taught by one professor she would have been given a passing grade on that assignment, but the same assignment would have earned a failing grade by a colleague professor teaching another section of the same course. How can we, as a profession, make sense of such a demonstrably unwarranted variance in grading of the same work? And the questions go on from there. How would we adjudicate a dispute between professor and student over a grade which seems on the evidence to be capricious or arbitrary? How would we advise the student to improve his or her work, when in fact the work stands as "excellent" in the eyes of some of us and as "failing" in the eyes of others of us?

To overcome our problem with divergent ratings, we discuss the reasons why the ratings were assigned. First the faculty talk together in pairs, then in groups of four, then the fours combine to make groups of eight. At each level of greater size, the faculty teams are asked to explain what they saw in the various student essays that led them to give it a particular score on the HCTSR. This is a critical thinking exercise in itself, where raters must reanalyze the essays, identifying the evidence justifying their judgment and explaining it to the other raters. It calls on the critical thinking skills of interpretation, analysis, evaluation, and explanation. It also calls for each participant to give fair-minded attention to the reasons others have for their divergent ratings, and to be willing to reconsider in light of the analyses being offered by others about the essay. If the faculty raters have strong critical thinking dispositions – and if they have not dominance structured, that is "dug in," around their preferred opinion – they can often hear what their colleagues are saying and at times be persuaded to change their scores. The practice of 'reason giving' is one that I hope they will generalize to other professional and life situations. Outliers may emerge, but in general there is a tendency toward consensus; this is particularly true when the faculty have generally evaluated a given essay as positive (4 or 3) or as negative (2 or 1). In this case, they usually gravitate toward one of the scores in each pair as their groups come to consensus regarding just how good or how bad the essay was.

The essay with ratings that range all the way from 4 to 1 at times defies ready consensus. Fundamentally the faculty have difficulty deciding simply whether it represents good critical thinking or poor critical thinking. This is in part because (a) the raters are still relatively inexperienced in talking with colleagues about their rating in any way whatsoever, or (b) they initially have difficulty explaining which specific aspects of a given piece of student work led them to form the judgment they have made. But the primary reason faculty disagree is because of (c) confounding critical thinking with other factors such as rhetorical style or writing quality. Students who use a lot of irony, sarcasm, or humor in writing their opinions seem to engender more polar responses in the faculty. And while it may be inappropriate for a variety of reasons to address the topic of genetic alteration of food with a Dennis Miller style rant in an academic context, that approach in and of itself does not make the critical thinking evidenced in the writing stronger or weaker. One must still make a rating of the rhetorical rant using the quality criteria outlined in the HCTSR. Similarly, poor grammar or composition must be ignored if the quality of the thinking being evidenced is strong. Thus, being able to parse out with precision those elements of the students' work that should or should not appropriately be considered when using the HCTSR, or in any other "grading" context, becomes a chief learning outcome of this lesson.

A second learning outcome I have for this exercise if that the faculty will come to understand that applying a rubric is like applying other abstract principles - such as promotion and tenure guidelines – we all understand what the guidelines mean by reference not only to the guidelines themselves but also by reference to the accumulated prior precedents. That is why sharing with students one's grading standards, as well as examples of the graded work of prior students, is an effective way to help the students understand where you "set the bar" for successful vs. unsuccessful work. With practiced use rubrics are internalized and, in the case of the HCTSR, we are soon able to identify a piece of work as characteristic of a '4,' quite distinct from another piece of work that would be rated a '2.' And more importantly, we become practiced at identifying significant evidence of the thinking process found in the essay and of providing our reasons for assigning the specific rating.

The third learning outcome intended by this workshop exercise with experienced colleagues is that they should come to appreciate the importance and the value of continuing collegial conversations regarding how the assignment of ratings and the evaluation of practice behavior requires the responsible explanation of how standards and guidelines are being applied in the classroom and the workplace. This becomes not only a matter of excellence in professional practice, but also a matter of justice and departmental responsibility and liability. In my judgment, to know that we disagree as faculty teaching alternative sections of the same course on whether a given piece of student work is a "pass" or a "fail" and not to address that disagreement in an objective, professional, informed, and fair-minded way is nothing short of irresponsible.

**Feedback from Participants**

I used this exercise with student work and the HCTST in workshops with faculty for over fifteen years and the reaction is always positive. Done with humor and respect, and with a willingness on all of our parts to "let the chips fall where they may," this exercise turns out to be both educational and enjoyable. I think it would be a more difficult exercise to use if the faculty were all from the same department, rather than the typical mix of people we find at national meetings. For one, they would have histories with one another, complex interpersonal and organizational relationships which began before the workshop and which must endure after the workshop. The lesson would have to be adapted, more precautions taken to assure that people can participate with minimal perceived risk to their long term collegial relationships, and more awareness that any given observation or comment comes with a potentially substantial amount of unspoken baggage. But, forty years in higher education, and much of that as chair, dean and provost, helps sensitize one to such things. And good colleagues realize that we should be able to talk in a fair-minded and collegially respectful way about our grading and performance ratings, not only for the sake of the health of our departments and programs, but also for the sake of the better educational development of our students and colleagues.

## Using the *Holistic Critical Thinking Scoring Rubric*

**1. Understand the construct:** This four level rubric treats critical thinking as a set of cognitive skills supported by certain personal dispositions. To reach a judicious, purposive judgment a good critical thinker engages in analysis, interpretation, evaluation, inference, explanation, and meta-cognitive self-regulation. The disposition to pursue fair-mindedly and open-mindedly the reasons and evidence wherever they lead is crucial to reaching sound, objective decisions and resolutions to complex, ill-structured problems. So are the other critical thinking dispositions, such as systematicity, reasoning self-confidence, cognitive maturity, analyticity, and inquisitiveness. [For details on the articulation of this concept refer to Critical Thinking: A Statement of Expert Consensus for Purposes of Educational Assessment and Instruction. ERIC Document Number: ED 315 423.]

**2. Differentiate and Focus**: Holistic scoring requires focus. In any essay, presentation, or clinical practice setting many elements must come together for overall success: critical thinking, content knowledge, and technical skill (craftsmanship). Deficits or strengths in any of these can draw the attention of the rater. However, in scoring for any one of the three, one must attempt to focus the evaluation on that element to the exclusion of the other two.

**3. Practice, Coordinate and Reconcile:** Ideally, in a training session with other raters one will examine sample essays (videotaped presentations, whatever is being evaluated) which are paradigmatic of each of the four levels. Without prior knowledge of their level, raters will be asked to evaluate and assign ratings to these samples. After comparing these preliminary ratings, collaborative analysis with the other raters and the trainer is used to achieve consistency of expectations among those who will be involved in rating the actual cases. Training, practice, and inter-rater reliability are the keys to a high quality assessment.

Usually, two raters will evaluate each essay, or assignment, or project, or performance. If they disagree there are three possible ways that resolution can be achieved: (a) by conversation between the two raters regarding their evaluations, (b) by using an independent third rater, or (c) by taking the average of the two initial ratings. The averaging strategy is strongly discouraged. Discrepancies between raters of more than one level suggest that detailed conversations about the CT construct and about project expectations are in order. This rubric is a four level scale, half point scoring is inconsistent with its intent and conceptual structure. Further, at this point in its history, the art and science of holistic critical thinking evaluation cannot justify asserting half-level differentiations.

When working alone, or without paradigm samples, one can achieve a greater level of internal consistency by not assigning final ratings until a number of essays, projects, assignments, performances have been viewed and given preliminary ratings. Frequently natural clusters or groupings of similar quality soon come to be discernible. At that point one can be more confident in assigning a firmer critical thinking score using this four level rubric. After assigning preliminary ratings, a review of the entire set assures greater internal consistency and fairness in the final ratings.

Download the HCTSR free from www.insightassessment.com/hctsr.html